Practical Diabetes Care

SECOND EDITION

Rowan Hillson, MD, FRCP
Consultant Physician
The Hillingdon Hospital

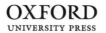

OXFORD
UNIVERSITY PRESS

OXFORD
UNIVERSITY PRESS

Great Clarendon Street, Oxford OX2 6DP

Oxford University Press is a department of the University of Oxford.
It furthers the University's objective of excellence in research, scholarship,
and education by publishing worldwide in

Oxford New York

Auckland Bangkok Buenos Aires Cape Town Chennai
Dar es Salaam Delhi Hong Kong Istanbul Karachi Kolkata
Kuala Lumpur Madrid Melbourne Mexico City Mumbai Nairobi
São Paulo Shanghai Taipei Tokyo Toronto

Oxford is a registered trade mark of Oxford University Press
in the UK and in certain other countries

Published in the United States
by Oxford University Press Inc., New York

© Rowan Hillson, 2002

The moral rights of the author have been asserted

Database right Oxford University Press (maker)

First edition published 1996
Second edition published 2002
Reprinted 2003

A catalogue record for this title is available from the British Library

Library of Congress Cataloging in Publication Data (Data available)

ISBN 0 19 263290 6 (Pbk)

10 9 8 7 6 5 4 3 2

Printed in Great Britain
on acid-free paper by T.J. International Ltd, Padstow

For Kay and Rodney Hillson

Diabetes is not a disease for specialists alone, not a disease solely for out-patient clinics with their medical personnel, but is *par excellence* a disease for interested family physicians to treat from its onset to its end throughout all the social, as well as physical, vicissitudes of patients' lives.

From Joslin, E.P., *et al.* (1947). *The treatment of diabetes.* Henry Plumpton, London.

Preface

In the year 2000 the International Diabetes Federation estimated that throughout the world about 4.6 per cent of all those aged 20 to 79 years had diabetes. That is about 150 million people worldwide. The figure for 1985 was 30 million; for 1995 it was 135 million. Diabetes is increasingly common. Some estimates suggest that there will be twice the number of people with diabetes in 2010 as there are now. However, it is also increasingly treatable, and possibly preventable by vigorous management of impairment of glucose tolerance.

Twenty-first century diabetes care has a substantial evidence base for practice. We now know that we can improve and probably lengthen our patients' lives by meticulous diabetes care, aiming to return the patient to as close to the non-diabetic state as possible. But treatment such as blood glucose normalization carries risks if not properly monitored. The patient will not feel you have improved his life if he has a bad hypoglycaemic attack and falls under a bus. However, the potential benefits of vigorous and carefully monitored treatment are considerable. All of this costs time and effort. Patients need to work harder at selfcare, staff need to provide more support. More patients are taking more drugs.

The challenge for everyone caring for people with diabetes is to find the best way of delivering evidence-based care to more and more patients in a friendly and practical way within limited resources. This means close co-operation between all concerned, with good communication and clear aims understood by all—particularly the patient.

This book includes information based on published studies and personal experience. It is not exhaustive; the body of diabetes literature is vast and growing daily. Ensure that your practice remains up to date by reading diabetes journals and attending educational diabetes meetings.

The Hillingdon Hospital   R. H.
2002

Preface to the first edition

This book is for general practitioners, practice nurses, dietitians, chiropodists, diabetes specialist nurses, and other general practice team members, working together to care for people who have diabetes. It will be particularly relevant for general practices establishing diabetic clinics, but each section also provides easily accessible guidelines for the management of 'one-off' diabetic problems. The book considers the problems patients bring to their diabetes advisers and practical ways of approaching and resolving them. Wherever possible emphasis is placed on helping the patients to help themselves, for our encounters with our patients are but brief intervals in their lives with diabetes.

For ease of reading the doctor is usually referred to as 'he' and other staff as 'she' throughout the text. Obviously doctors may be female (as I am) and nurses, for example, may be male, and no insult is intended to the opposite sex. The chapters are illustrated by case histories. These are based on real patients but details have been altered, or histories combined, to protect patient confidentiality. Throughout 'diabetes' means diabetes mellitus unless specified otherwise.

Hillingdon   R. H.
September 1995

Acknowledgements

Over the years many people have shared their knowledge and enthusiasm for diabetes with me—people with diabetes, my teachers in medicine, and my colleagues in hospital medicine and in general practice. I thank you all.

I am especially grateful to Professor Philip Home, consultant diabetologist and recent editor of *Diabetic Medicine*, and Dr Robert Asher, general practitioner, for reading the draft manuscript, and for their detailed and constructive comments.

I also wish to thank Mrs Gill Ruane, Mrs Brenda Cox, the Hillingdon Diabetes Team, Mr and Mrs W.R. Hillson, and the staff at Oxford University Press for their support and contributions to the project.

Tables 7.1 and 9.2 are reproduced from MIMS with kind permission of Colin Duncan. (These tables are updated every month in MIMS). Table 18.2 is reproduced from Table 32 of the *Manual of nutrition* (1985) with permission of the Controller of Her Majesty's Stationery Office. Material included in pp. 124–9 is reproduced by kind permission of Kluwer Academic Publishers, from *Diabetic eye disease* by E. Kritzinger and K. Taylor (1984). The St Vincent Declaration (p. 205) as published in *Diabetic Medicine*, (1990), 7, p. 360, is reproduced by permission of the International Diabetes Federation, Europe, Professor H. Krans, and John Wiley and Sons Ltd. The European Patients' Charter (p. 206) as published in *Diabetic Medicine*, (1991), 8, 782–3, is reproduced by permission of the International Diabetes Federation, Europe, Professor K.G.M.M. Alberti, and John Wiley and Sons Ltd. The following figures are taken from books by Dr Rowan Hillson with permission from Little, Brown & Co (UK) Ltd p. 2 (*Diabetes: a young person's guide*), pp. 87, 88, 89 (*Diabetes: a new guide*), p. 117 (*Diabetes: a beyond basics guide*). Sections of the Hillingdon Consensus Care Diabetes Project Guidelines are reproduced with the kind permission of the Consensus Care Group.

Contents

Chapter 1

The path to diagnosis

Diabetes presents in many forms to different people in different fields. The person to whom it presents or the place in which it is diagnosed affects the initial assessment and management. The general practitioner is the central and constant figure in the patient's care. Once you suspect the diagnosis of diabetes, confirm it, tell the patient the diagnosis, and explain what happens next.

Presentations

Patients may seek help with the classical symptoms of hyperglycaemia, symptoms of diabetic tissue damage, or those of conditions causing diabetes. Some patients may present with symptoms not usually associated with diabetes but glycosuria or hyperglycaemia may be found as part of routine screening. Other people, who believe themselves to be well, undergo physical and biochemical examination for employment, insurance purposes, or health screening (Table 1.1).

The way in which the diagnosis comes to light influences the patient's attitude to his or her condition. Those with thirst and polyuria want relief from their symptoms and may be more likely to comply with treatment than those patients who feel well.

Table 1.1 The path to diagnosis of diabetes

Patient-initiated

Symptoms of hyperglycaemia (e.g. thirst, polyuria)
Symptoms of diabetic tissue damage
Symptoms of conditions causing diabetes (e.g. steroid excess)
Unrelated symptoms leading to general biochemical screen

Screening

Well-person health check (state decreed or patient request)
Insurance medical
Employment medical
During training in glucose testing (e.g. nurse)

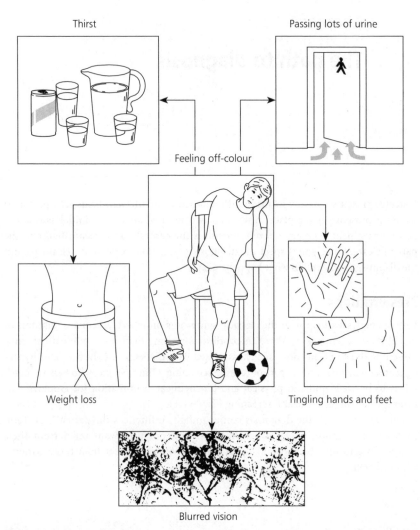

Thirst

Passing lots of urine

Feeling off-colour

Weight loss

Tingling hands and feet

Blurred vision

Fig. 1.1 Symptoms of diabetes

Symptoms of diabetes (Fig. 1.1)

Thirst, polydipsia, and polyuria

The thirst of untreated diabetes is not easily slaked. Unfortunately many people choose sucrose or glucose-rich aerated drinks like lemonade or cola which temporarily relieve the thirst but exacerbate the underlying problem. At night they will have a glass of water on the bedside table. A few people, often elderly, are sufficiently strong-willed to ignore their thirst for fear of increasing their polyuria. This leads to severe dehydration and may precipitate hospital admission.

Polyuria is the frequent passage of large volumes of urine. The urine is usually virtually colourless. The patient may be wakened at night by the need to micturate. Teresa McLean (1985) said 'It is hard to describe how enervating it was to get up six or seven times a night to pee. I was living in a bed-sit in London and used to lie in bed at night and pray for one, just, one, night of unbroken sleep, then wake up to pee again.' In children or elderly people nocturnal polyuria may manifest itself as urinary incontinence. People with or without pre-existing sphincter problems may suffer daytime stress incontinence or bedwetting. The development of diabetes in men with prostatism may precipitate urinary retention. Although the thirst and polydipsia are secondary to the polyuria, some patients deny polyuria whilst bitterly complaining of thirst. Some of them assume that the large volumes of urine are secondary to their increased fluid intake and are therefore unworthy of comment.

Logically, the degree of hyperglycaemia should determine the amount of glycosuria, the severity of the polyuria, and hence the thirst and polydipsia. However, this is not necessarily so and symptoms are a poor guide to the patient's blood glucose concentration, not least because degrees of stoicism and personal observation vary. Polyuria without glycosuria is not due to diabetes mellitus and other causes must be sought (see p. 11).

Weight loss

Aretaeos the Cappadocian believed that the body tissues melted away into the urine—a supposition not far from the modern view. Some of the weight loss is due to dehydration—the rest to reduction of adipose tissue by lipolysis and muscle breakdown to fuel gluconeogenesis. The obese patient may be overjoyed at her weight loss, not realizing that this is a manifestation of a disease process soon to be diagnosed as diabetes. After initiation of treatment her lost weight may be regained. Classically, the weight loss of diabetes mellitus is associated with a normal or even increased appetite. A few patients crave sweet foods. Cachexia may develop rapidly in patients with insulin-dependent diabetes (Type 1 diabetes) who were slim to start with or in whom the diagnosis has been delayed. Many patients with non-insulin dependent diabetes (Type 2 diabetes) do not lose weight and in patients with steroid-induced diabetes the weight gain of steroid excess may balance the weight loss of untreated diabetes.

Tiredness and malaise

Tiredness is an insidious but frequent symptom. It ranges from a slight dampening of *joie de vivre* to exhaustion and inability to work. 'Even when the pressure was on I couldn't produce. I was finding it just a drag to get out of bed . . . I was literally falling asleep in meetings. It was awful!' (Gwyn: Maclean and Oram 1988). Non-specific malaise may be unnoticed until the treated patient looks back in retrospect. Their friends and family may complain that the patient is irritable and hard to live with.

Bowel symptoms

Dehydration may cause constipation as more water than usual is absorbed from the faeces. In the elderly diabetes may present as severe constipation. A few patients have the pale, offensive, loose stools of steatorrhoea due to pancreatic disease reducing both enzyme and hormone production.

Recurrent or refractory infections

Some people with diabetes seek medical help because of boils or other skin infections. Some of these patients may be nasal carriers of *Staphylococcus aureus*. Others may have recurrent fungal infections such as moniliasis despite anti-fungal therapy. Glycosuria should be sought in all women with thrush and men with balanitis. Recurrent urinary tract or chest infections may also presage diabetes.

Visual disturbance

Changes in blood glucose concentrations may alter the refractive index of the lens, aqueous humour, and cornea and cause blurred vision. Patients may visit their optician and leave with a prescription for expensive new spectacles which may be useless once the hyperglycaemia resolves. However, some new diagnoses of diabetes are made by opticians. Additional symptoms relating to tissue damage are discussed below.

Paraesthesiae

Pins and needles are felt in hands and feet and usually resolve on treatment of the diabetes. In some patients they represent permanent peripheral nerve damage which may persist or worsen.

Pruritus

Pruritus vulvae is a common presenting feature, due to candidal infection. Generalized pruritus is not a feature of diabetes alone—seek pancreatic malignancy or other serious pathology.

Cramp

Patients with uncontrolled diabetes often complain of cramp, especially in the legs, probably secondary to diuresis. If persistent it can be relieved by quinine sulphate.

Symptoms of diabetes tissue damage

These will be discussed in the relevant sections below. Diabetes can remain undetected for many years and its first manifestation may be a myocardial infarction or a foot ulcer.

No symptoms

It is estimated that about half the patients with diabetes in the community remained undetected. Some may be ignoring symptoms (Tables 1.1 and 1.2) but others appear genuinely asymptomatic—12 per cent of patients with Type 2 diabetes in one study (Hillson *et al.* 1985).

There is increasing evidence that diabetic tissue damage begins long before diabetes is actually diagnosed. Thirty-five per cent of patients with newly recognized Type 2

Table 1.2 Symptoms of diabetes

General

Thirst and polydipsia
Polyuria
Weight loss
Tiredness, malaise, irritability
Constipation
Visual disturbance (e.g. blurring)
Paraesthesiae
Pruritus
Cramp
Repeated or slow-healing infections, especially skin

Tissue damage

Any form of tissue damage may present. Commoner ones are:
Ischaemic heart disease
Peripheral vascular disease
Cerebrovascular disease
Neuropathy
Cataract or retinal disease

Conditions causing diabetes

Steroid excess (iatrogenic) is the commonest

diabetes (see p. 10) have tissue damage already. Diabetes UK used data from an audit of 155 000 patients with Type 2 diabetes to perform linear regression analysis to calculate the number of years before diagnosis that small vessel complications (and hence diabetes) began to occur. The audit suggested a 10-year delay in diagnosing diabetes (Diabetes UK 2000). However it also indicated that large vessel complications started 20 years before diagnosis. This is consistent with the known link between impaired glucose tolerance (see p. 8) and cardiovascular disease. It seems highly likely that people with diabetes progress from impaired fasting glucose and/or impaired glucose tolerance to frank diabetes over a period of years. It is only the latter state which may produce symptoms. It is therefore essential that we identify patients with all degrees of glucose intolerance as early as possible to allow risk reduction care.

Screening

'Well-person' screening usually includes urine glucose testing; however, some people with diabetes do not have glycosuria. A post-prandial urine sample is more likely to detect diabetes. Twenty-two per cent of those with diabetes identified in one study had post-prandial glycosuria but no glucose in a fasting sample (Davies *et al.* 1991). Blood glucose estimations may also be used for screening but great care should be used in large-scale finger-prick screening campaigns (Table 1.3).

Table 1.3 Who should be screened for diabetes?

Screen every 3 years (at least)

Those with symptoms of diabetes

Those presenting with tissue damage known to be associated with diabetes

Those with conditions known to cause or to be associated with diabetes (e.g. many endocrinopathies)

Those on medication known to be associated with diabetes (e.g. steroids, thiazides)

Pregnant women (see p. 164)

First-degree adult relatives of non-insulin treated patients

Patients over 60 years old

Asian and Afro-Caribbean patients

Obese patients (especially if abdominal)

Patients with a family history of ischaemic heart disease

A 10-year-old boy was brought to a diabetes information stand at a county show. A voluntary screening group had just diagnosed diabetes on the basis of a finger-prick glucose level of 11.5 mmol/l. His distraught mother, clutching a large, sticky lolly, begged for help. On questioning, the boy tearfully admitted that the lolly was his—confiscated because 'diabetics can't eat sweets.' After a thorough hand wash his finger-prick glucose was 4 mmol/l.

Screening by random finger-prick or venous blood glucose testing can be difficult to interpret. It is quick and simple and can be used for opportunistic screening but unfortunately creates a large pool of 'diabetes uncertain' patients.

Making the diagnosis

The diagnosis of diabetes has major implications for the individual, not only as regards changes in lifestyle and the introduction of self-monitoring and medication, but also with regard to employment, insurance, driving, sports, and hobbies. It is therefore essential to prove the diagnosis at the outset.

The diagnostic criteria for diabetes changed in June 2000. You can use finger-prick glucose tests in the surgery but the formal diagnosis can only be made on venous

Finger-prick glucose over 9.5 mmol/l:

Send a venous plasma glucose now, except in child or ill adult

- Child—refer to hospital same day
- Ill adult—refer to hospital same day

Finger-prick glucose 5–9.5 mmol/l:

Do **fasting** venous plasma glucose

- Fasting venous plasma glucose below 6 mmol/l—normal
- Fasting venous plasma glucose 6–7 mmol/l—IFG; do OGTT
- Fasting venous plasma glucose over 7 mmol/l—diabetes

plasma glucose samples. Finger-prick systems may use whole blood which gives lower results. Venous samples should also be used if there is any uncertainty about a finger-prick result or there is a high likelihood of diabetes clinically. (One sample if diabetic symptoms, two samples without symptoms.) You may need to do a 75 g oral glucose tolerance test (OGTT) (see Table 1.4) to find out whether the patient has diabetes or impaired glucose tolerance (IGT) (see Table 1.5 (a)). Impaired fasting glucose (IFG) is a new category (see Table 1.5 (b)). If you have a clear diagnosis of diabetes on one (or two) venous laboratory glucose samples, or if the patient is known to be diabetic, there is no need to do an OGTT.

Each practice should develop a diabetes screening policy which is practical for their surgery and their patients. One option is to test for urine glucose in every new attender, and in every patient over 40, once a year or opportunistically. In patients at higher risk of diabetes (see Table 1.3) perform a random blood glucose test if the patient has diabetic symptoms or signs of diabetic tissue damage, and in those who are poor attenders. Otherwise measure fasting glucose.

Table 1.4(a) The oral glucose tolerance test (75 g)

1. Ask the patient to eat his/her normal diet. If the dietary carbohydrate is less than 125 g daily, the patient should eat 150 g daily for the three days before the test.
2. Fast the patient overnight for 10–14 hours. He/she should eat nothing, drink only water, and should not smoke during this time nor during the test.
3. The patient should be sitting at rest during the test.
4. Take a venous blood sample for plasma glucose estimation. Test the urine for glucose.
5. Give the patient 75 g glucose dissolved in 250–350 ml water to be swallowed over 5–15 minutes. (Lucozade can be used.)
6. Two hours after the start of the test take another venous blood sample for plasma glucose estimation. Test the urine for glucose.
7. Ensure all samples are labelled with the patient's name, the time, and the date. Ensure that the request card(s) mirrors this labelling.

Table 1.4(b) Interpreting the results of the oral glucose tolerance test

	Venous plasma glucose concentration (mmol/l)		
	Fasting		2 hours after glucose load
Diabetes	≥7.0	OR	≥11.1
Impaired glucose tolerance	<7.0	AND	7.8–11.0
Impaired fasting glucose	6–6.9	AND	<11.1

Table 1.5(a) Impaired glucose tolerance (IGT)

OGTT: Fasting venous plasma glucose below 7 mmol/l
        Two-hour venous plasma glucose 7.8–11.0 mmol/l

Not a benign condition

This condition is associated with a substantial risk of future diabetes (about 10 per cent per annum). In overweight people appropriate diet and exercise greatly reduce the risk of developing diabetes. IGT is also associated with increased risk of cardiovascular disease.

Check for cardiovascular disease—heart, brain, peripheries

Check and treat risk factors

Smoking
Blood pressure
Weight
Lack of exercise
Fasting cholesterol (total, HDL, LDL)
Triglyceride

Tell the patient...

'Your body is not using glucose properly. You do not have diabetes although this condition may lead to diabetes. Healthy eating, so your weight is normal for your height, with regular exercise will reduce your risk of developing diabetes.' Give them a copy of their results. Explain the risk of diabetes and heart and circulatory disease (and what both of these are). Warn the patient to seek a blood glucose test if they experience thirst, increased urination, weight loss, thrush/perineal irritation, undue tiredness; or if they are ill, injured, or pregnant.

Recheck fasting glucose

Venous plasma glucose at OGTT <6 mmol/l—recheck it annually, repeat OGTT if 6–7 mmol/l
Venous plasma glucose at OGTT 6–7 mmol/l—follow impaired fasting glucose pathway

This guideline was adapted by the author from the Diabetes UK Guidelines of June 2000, with the help of Dr Dai Thomas, The Hillingdon Hospital.

Table 1.5(b) Impaired fasting glucose (IFG)

OGTT: Fasting venous plasma glucose 6–7 mmol/l
        Two-hour venous plasma glucose below 11.1 mmol/l

This new category identifies people likely to develop diabetes. Patients can have both IFG and impaired glucose tolerance (IGT) and such patients have a high risk of diabetes and should be followed closely.

Check for cardiovascular disease—heart, brain, peripheries

Check and treat risk factors

Smoking
Blood pressure
Weight

Lack of exercise
Fasting cholesterol (total, HDL, LDL)
Triglyceride

Tell the patient...

'Your blood sugar is higher than normal but not in the diabetic range. You may develop diabetes although this process can be slowed by early treatment.' Explain what diabetes is. Give the patient a copy of their results. Warn the patient to seek a blood glucose test if they experience thirst, increased urination, weight loss, thrush/perineal irritation, undue tiredness; or if they are ill, injured, or pregnant.

Recheck fasting glucose

Recheck fasting venous plasma glucose in three months; then every six months
If IFG *and* IGT, check every three months, longterm
If IFG persists do an OGTT annually

Consensus awaited

IFG is a new category of glucose intolerance. The patient cannot be officially diagnosed as diabetic until he/she has a fasting glucose over 7.0 mmol/l or a two-hour glucose above 11.0 mmol/l.

This guideline was adapted by the author from the Diabetes UK Guidelines of June 2000, with the help of Dr Dai Thomas, The Hillingdon Hospital.

Metabolic stress

In patients whose blood glucose levels suggest diabetes but who are under meta-bolic stress such as an infection, myocardial infarction, surgery, or a course of steroid treatment, repeat the blood glucose tests at least six weeks after the patient has recov-ered to confirm the persistence of diabetes. A glycosylated haemoglobin reading may be helpful—if raised the patient is highly likely to have diabetes.

Ill patients

Do not delay treatment of severely hyperglycaemic and clinically ill patients because laboratory confirmation is unobtainable or slow. If the finger-prick glucose concentra-tion is over 25 mmol/l wash another of the patient's fingers with plain water, dry well, and repeat the finger-prick glucose. If hyperglycaemia is confirmed treat the patient accordingly, but send a pre-treatment blood sample to the laboratory for blood glucose estimation.

Pregnancy

Many authorities consider that these diagnostic criteria also apply to pregnant women. However, different criteria are sometimes used in pregnancy (see p. 164).

Retrospective diagnosis of diabetes

Occasionally, a doctor is presented with a patient in whom oral hypoglycaemic treat-ment for diabetes has already been started without proper confirmation of the diagnosis.

This should not occur if the guidelines above are followed. If the patient is seen within six weeks of starting medication, the finding of a raised haemoglobin $A1_c$ (p. 62) provides support for the diagnosis of diabetes. Sometimes the oral hypoglycaemic treatment has to be stopped to allow clarification of the diagnosis.

Types of diabetes

Type 1 and Type 2 diabetes

The same blood glucose criteria apply to the diagnosis of all types of diabetes. The two main types are Type 1 (insulin-dependent diabetes or juvenile-onset diabetes previously) and Type 2 (non-insulin-dependent or maturity-onset diabetes previously).

People with Type 1 diabetes are usually:

◆ under 40 years of age

◆ slim

◆ ketosis-prone

◆ islet-cell antibody positive

◆ have rapid onset of symptoms (often severe)

◆ unable to survive without insulin treatment

People with Type 2 diabetes are usually:

◆ over 40 years of age

◆ overweight

◆ not ketosis-prone

◆ islet-cell antibody negative

◆ have variable onset of symptoms (often slow and less severe)

◆ able to survive without insulin treatment

A subset of people with Type 2 diabetes have maturity-onset diabetes of the young (MODY). This usually starts under 25 years of age and forms 2–5 per cent of Type 2 diabetes. Fifty per cent of parents and 50 per cent of siblings have glucose intolerance; it is slowly progressive and seldom needs insulin. Various gene defects have been identified. Early-onset Type 2 diabetes starts between 25 and 40 years of age. Ninety per cent of parents and 68 per cent of siblings have glucose intolerance. It is associated with obesity. Insulin is often needed and microvascular complications are common. (Rehman 2001)

Some patients are difficult to classify but can still be treated on clinical and biochemical assessment. Tropical diabetes is not seen in Britain and is associated with pancreatic calculi and, in some instances, with malnutrition.

Secondary diabetes

Drugs such as thiazides and other diuretics (especially in combination with beta blockers), and steroids are the commonest cause of secondary diabetes. Other rare causes are alcoholic pancreatic disease and other pancreatitis, acromegaly, Cushing's syndrome, thyrotoxicosis, haemochromatosis, phaeochromocytoma, glucagonoma, and treated thalassaemia. The patient with jaundice or abdominal pain may have carcinoma of the pancreas.

Non-diabetic conditions

Differential diagnosis

Prostatism causes urinary frequency. Hypercalcaemia may cause polyuria and polydipsia. Rarely thirst, polyuria, and polydipsia are due to insufficiency of antidiuretic hormone—diabetes insipidus. There is nearly always a history of pituitary disease, head injury, or intracranial or other features suggestive of endocrinopathy. Very rarely, both diabetes mellitus and diabetes insipidus occur together as part of the hereditary DIDMOAD syndrome (diabetes insipidus, diabetes mellitus, optic atrophy, and deafness) or in patients with acromegaly or Cushing's disease whose tumour or its surgical treatment have induced antidiuretic hormone deficiency. Compulsive water drinking can also produce these symptoms.

Renal glycosuria

This is due to a low renal threshold for glucose allowing glucose to spill into the urine at normal blood glucose levels. This is rare and usually inherited. It is very important to document accurately. Ensure that the patient and his/her general practitioner have a copy of the results. Such patients suffer much frustration at being repeatedly labelled diabetic in insurance examinations, employment medicals, or by doctors unfamiliar with their case. Make sure that the patient understands what is going on and that they learn the term renal glycosuria. Of course, by coincidence, a few such patients become diabetic in later years. If they have symptoms of diabetes the blood glucose concentration should be measured.

Summary

- Diabetes may present with thirst, polydipsia, polyuria, weight loss, visual disturbance, or paraesthesiae. A random venous plasma glucose concentration of 11.1 mmol/l or more or a fasting venous plasma glucose of 7.0 mmol/l or above confirms the diagnosis.

- In asymptomatic patients, glycosuria may suggest the diagnosis. It must be confirmed by two random venous plasma glucose concentrations of 11.1 mmol/l or more, or two fasting venous plasma glucose levels of 7.0 mmol/l or more, or a combination of random and fasting glucose levels.

- Tell the patient what you have found and if they have diabetes, what this means.

References and further reading

Davies, M., Alban-Davies, H., Cook, C., and Day, J. (1991). Self-testing for diabetes mellitus. *British Medical Journal*, **303**, 696–8.

Diabetes UK. (2000) Audit shows 10-year delay in diagnosing diabetes. *Diabetes update*, **23**, 1–3.

Hillson, R.M., Hockaday, T.D.R., Newton, D.J., and Pim, B. (1985). Delayed diagnosis of NIDDM is associated with greater metabolic and clinical abnormality. *Diabetic Medicine*, **2**, 383–8.

Maclean, H., and Oram, B. (1988). *Living with diabetes*. University of Toronto Press, Toronto.

McLean, T. (1985). *Metal jam. The story of a diabetic*. Hodder & Stoughton, London.

Neil, H.A.W., Gatling, W., Mather, H.M., Thompson, A.V., Thorogood, M., Fowler, G.H., *et al.* (1987). The Oxford Community Diabetes Study: evidence for an increase in the prevalence of known diabetes in Great Britain. *Diabetic Medicine*, **4**, 539–43.

Rehman, H.U. (2001). Diabetes mellitus in the young. *Journal of the Royal Society of Medicine*, **94**, 65–7.

Skarfors, E.T., Selinus, K.I., and Lithell, H.O. (1991). *British Medical Journal*, **303**, 755–60.

World Health Organisation (1985). WHO study group. *Diabetes mellitus*. WHO Technical Report Series 727.

Chapter 2

The first steps

This chapter assumes that the patient has newly-proven diabetes mellitus. Once the diagnosis has been made assess the patient thoroughly, teach him or her about diabetes, and initiate treatment. If the patient is referred to a diabetic clinic without adequate proof of diagnosis this must be obtained first. Each person with diabetes should be cared for by professionals trained and experienced in diabetes management, in close liaison with other carers. Unless the general practice team has this expertise, refer new patients to a diabetologist. Subsequent care can then be agreed as appropriate. Patients aged under 20 years should always be referred to a specialist diabetes team same day.

Referring the new patient to a diabetic clinic

Urgent or non-urgent referral?

Patients with untreated Type 1 diabetes should be assessed and treated promptly as they can decompensate rapidly. If in doubt telephone the diabetologist to discuss the patient.

> Karen and her husband are South African and in their mid-twenties. They came to Britain with dysentery after a world tour. Her husband recovered but Karen did not. The diarrhoea disappeared but she was very thirsty, had polyuria, continued weight loss, and felt terrible. One Friday a doctor diagnosed diabetes, referred Karen to a diabetic clinic and told her to wait for the appointment. No further action was taken. By Monday Karen felt very ill. In desperation she boarded a plane for South Africa and her previous family doctor. He started her on insulin and she improved rapidly. On her return to Britain she found an appointment to attend a diabetic clinic—three weeks after her initial diagnosis.

Urgent (that is, same day) referral

Patients with any of the following features usually warrant admission:
- a child
- any impairment of conscious level or confusion
- clinically ill
- vomiting
- hyperventilation
- severe dehydration
- low blood pressure

Urgent (that is, same day) referral *(continued)*

- fever
- foot or leg infection or gangrene
- blood glucose over 25 mmol/l (some patients tolerate high glucose levels well but it may be difficult to decide who needs urgent help and who can be managed at home)
- patients with concomitant severe illness, especially infection.

Consider giving adults 4–10 units fast-acting insulin subcutaneously (s.c.) (intramuscularly (i.m.) if shocked) immediately if the diagnosis of diabetes is secure.

Patients with any of these features may not need admission but do need urgent assessment:

- severe symptoms
- profuse urinary ketones
- marked weight loss
- under 30 years of age

Consider giving adults 4–10 units fast-acting insulin s.c. immediately if the diagnosis of diabetes is secure.

Assessing a person with diabetes—information needed by the diabetes care team

Demographic and practical

In addition to the usual information (patient's name, address, telephone number, date of birth, and hospital or record number if relevant):

- current occupation(s)
- language spoken if not English: the name and telephone number of an interpreter
- hearing, visual, speech, or other communication problems
- comprehension problems (e.g. Down's syndrome)
- mobility problems or other physical disabilities
- religious or other beliefs which may influence treatment (e.g. vegetarian, non-beef eating, non-pork eating, no blood products, clothing taboos).

Clinical history

Presentation of diabetes The duration of symptoms prior to diagnosis is very variable—in one study a patient had experienced thirst for 14 years before diagnosis. Symptom duration is an approximate guide to the minimum duration of diabetes. Prolonged symptoms before diagnosis is, not surprisingly, linked with increased likelihood of tissue damage. Symptoms are detailed in Table 1.2 (p. 5).

Previous medical history Relevant features to identify are those suggestive of large or small vessel disease, for example myocardial infarction or renal disease; endocrine disorders such as hypothyroidism; or other autoimmune disorders such as pernicious anaemia. Have there been conditions likely to require steroid treatment or diuretics? Previous obstetric history, in particular the birth of large babies, is also important.

Family history Seek that of diabetes and arterial disease, and other endocrinopathy or autoimmune disorder.

Social history This is one of the most important and neglected parts of the history.

Education When did the patient leave school? Has he or she had any further education? Everyone with diabetes needs to understand his or her condition and how to care for themselves—this information must be conveyed in a way which the patient can understand.

Occupation Ascertain details of the patient's occupation—is he a shift worker, working with machinery, driving, travelling frequently, doing a physically strenuous job? Would he be at serious risk of injury if hypoglycaemia occurred at work? Can people with diabetes hold this particular job—for example, insulin-treated patients are not allowed to drive passenger carrying vehicles. The diagnosis may have important financial implications.

Family circle and dependents Is the patient living alone or with support of family or friends?

Accommodation Does the patient live in a house or flat, with or without stairs? Is he/she in a nursing home or warden-supervised accommodation?

Leisure activities Are these energetic activities such as football, athletics, martial arts, or potentially hazardous activities like sky diving or underwater diving. Enquire about the level of other physical activity and less active hobbies requiring good eyesight like needlework, painting, or reading.

Smoking habits Many Asian patients do not smoke cigarettes and may not consider the hookah or bindi as smoking.

Alcohol intake If excessive in the past, the patient could have diabetes secondary to chronic pancreatitis. If excessive now, weight and triglycerides may rise and there is a risk of hypoglycaemia with glucose-lowering medication (see p. 104).

Drugs and allergies Patients should bring all their drugs to every clinic appointment. Steroids, oral contraceptive preparations, and thiazides worsen insensitivity to insulin and may precipitate hyperglycaemia. Beta blockers may reduce warning of hypoglycaemia and worsen the lipid profile. Allergy to sulphonamides precludes treatment with sulphonylurea drugs.

Direct questions or systemic inquiry These should not be skimped. Positive answers may indicate tissue damage. Other disorders can produce problems with diabetes, for example a patient with prostatism may develop urinary retention with marked polyuria.

Blood glucose concentration(s) Obtained by any referring doctor and whether fasting or non-fasting. Is the diagnosis proven? If not, what is the diagnosis?

Clinical examination

Perform a full clinical examination. Factors especially relevant to diabetes are the acute consequences of hyperglycaemia, tissue damage, and evidence of conditions causing secondary diabetes or associated with diabetes. The detailed section below includes some uncommon findings for completeness. Examples of abnormalities which may be found in diabetes are given but there may obviously be many other causes for some signs. The details of diabetic tissue damage are discussed in Chapter 13.

State of consciousness

Impaired conscious level necessitates urgent consideration of diabetic ketoacidosis or of a non-ketotic severely hyperglycaemic state. Remember that there is a high frequency of cerebrovascular disease and hence strokes in people with diabetes.

Personality/psychological features

The patient's personality and attitudes will influence his capability to cope with the diagnosis of diabetes and his ability to manage his own care. An impression of his or her approach to this first interview helps to assess the degree and rate of diabetes teaching and the degree of responsibility given to the patient at this and later stages.

General observations

During the examination be alert for clues to secondary diabetes, including alcoholic pancreatic disease, acromegaly, thyrotoxicosis, Cushing's syndrome, haemochromatosis, phaeochromocytoma. Patients with congenital rubella may have heart disease, cataracts, and deafness. However, most patients will have diabetes alone.

Weight and height

Assessment of weight in relation to height is essential. Type 1 patients may be underweight. Those with Type 2 diabetes often have abdominal obesity which may also be associated with hypertension, hypertriglyceridaemia, and cardiovascular disease (Reaven's syndrome).

Skin

Skin infections (boils, cellulitis, ulcers, fungi) are common. Less common signs include diabetic dermopathy, necrobiosis lipoidica diabeticorum (p. 134), and granuloma annulare. Some patients have vitiligo as a marker of autoimmune disease. A jaundiced patient may have a pancreatic malignancy. Sweating may be reduced in autonomic neuropathy.

Seek stigmata of hyperlipidaemia (p. 136)—xanthelasmata or corneal arcus, xanthomata elsewhere, and fatty deposition in tendons (for example, hands or Achilles tendon).

Infection Common in people with diabetes. Seek fever or lymph node enlargement.

Dehydration May be severe in those patients with marked hyperglycaemia.

Thyroid Enlargement should be sought as thyroid disease may be associated with diabetes.

Cardiovascular system

In addition to examining the pulse, venous pressure, apex, heart sounds, and seeking oedema, measure both lying and standing blood pressure and take particular note of lower limb pulses. Abnormal findings in people with diabetes may include the following:

1 hypertension: common in people with diabetes

2 postural hypotension: autonomic neuropathy, severe dehydration

3 hypotension: cardiac disease, severe dehydration

4 left ventricular hypertrophy: hypertension

5 mid-systolic aortic murmur: aortic sclerosis

6 pansystolic apical murmur: mitral regurgitation after myocardial infarct

7 peripheral pulses reduced or missing: peripheral vascular disease (see foot and leg examination)

8 ankle or sacral oedema: cardiac failure, nephrotic syndrome

Respiratory system

As usual note the rate and character of respiration, sputum, chest expansion, percussion note, and breath sounds. Abnormal findings in people with diabetes may include the following:

1 Kussmaul respiration (hyperventilation or air hunger): ketoacidosis, renal failure

2 chest infection: common in diabetes

3 asthma or chronic airflow limitation treated with steroids

Abdomen

Abdominal examination for tenderness, masses, and organomegaly is usually normal but genital examination often reveals thrush. People with diabetes may show:

Hepatomegaly: haemochromatosis; sometimes in alcoholic liver disease. Splenomegaly may be due to portal hypertension

Kidneys: tender or enlarged (consider infection, abscess); renal bruits (arteriopaths)

Pancreatic mass: an uncommon sign of pancreatic tumour

Genitalia: balanitis or pruritus vulvi (fungal infections)

Nervous system

Ophthalmic examination is mandatory as is a search for peripheral neuropathy. The detail in which the rest of the nervous system is examined obviously depends on symptoms.

Eyes Examine visual acuity, eye movements, lenses, and fundi (see p. 124). Reduced visual acuity is a late sign of diabetic eye disease

Ophthalmoplegia: diabetic mononeuropathy

Cataract: common in diabetes

Retinopathy: common

Hearing Should be assessed. Deafness impairs education unless recognized and may be due to diabetic tissue damage.

Cranial nerves Seek evidence of stroke or diabetic mononeuropathy.

Limbs Seek evidence of diabetic neuropathy or stroke (see foot and leg examination, p. 146). Always test tendon reflexes and observe gait.

Joints and ligaments

Always examine hand and foot joints (and other joints in which there are symptoms).
Dupuytren's contracture: associated with diabetes
Cheiroarthropathy (p. 134); also hammer or claw toes
Charcot joints (pp. 135, 147)

Arthritic changes may make insulin injection or finger-prick glucose testing difficult. Patients treated with steroids for severe arthritis may have steroid-induced diabetes.

Feet

These may have been included in other systems although it is usually simpler to check the following together at the end of the examination:

- foot hygiene
- previous surgery or amputation
- skin condition
- pressure areas
- blemishes—cracks, blisters
- old or current ulcers
- deformities
- circulation—cutaneous and pulses
- sensation—especially pin-prick, position, and vibration
- shoes

Comment

To see a patient in this depth takes 30 to 60 minutes. Skimping here may lead to repetition and time-wasting later. It should be remembered that the majority of people with newly diagnosed diabetes do not have other endocrinopathies. However, it is important not to miss clues to conditions which require their own different treatment which may, in turn, improve the diabetes. A further point is that many 'new' diabetic patients, especially elderly people, already have evidence of large or small blood vessel disease. In some instances this is severe enough to warrant urgent treatment (for example, laser photocoagulation, treatment of foot ulcer).

What now?

Summarize what you have found in the medical record. As you do so, build yourself a mental picture of the person, his diabetes, and how it has affected him. Plan the management and treatment.

Tell the patient what you have found (if you have found nothing abnormal on examination say so). With constant reference to the patient, plan further investigations and agree the management and treatment. There may be only one option, but it is more acceptable to the patient if he or she has worked it through with you.

Further investigations

Height and weight Aim for a body mass index (weight (kg)/height^2 (m^2)) between 18 and 25. Use a growth chart for patients under 19 years old.

Urine tests Urine glucose, ketones, and protein. Request microscopy and culture if there is proteinuria or symptoms of urinary tract infection or renal disease.

Blood tests

- random venous plasma glucose, haemoglobin A1$_c$, or fructosamine
- full blood count
- creatinine, sodium, potassium
- cholesterol and triglyceride (preferably fasting, see p. 136)
- liver function tests
- thyroid function tests (and other endocrine tests if indicated)

Electrocardiogram In patients with hypertension or signs or symptoms suggesting cardiac disease. (Some doctors would perform an ECG in most patients with Type 2 diabetes.)

Chest X-ray In smokers, hypertensive patients, those with evidence of respiratory or cardiac disease, and those from tuberculosis-prone populations.

What type of diabetes?

Type 1 diabetes

- Under 40 years old
- Thin or marked weight loss
- Ketotic
- Rapid onset of symptoms (often severe)

Type 2 diabetes

- Over 40 years old
- Overweight
- Not markedly ketotic
- Variable onset of symptoms (often slow and less severe)

Note that some under-30s may have Type 2 and that many Type 2 patients may eventually need insulin. Type 1 diabetes can occur in the elderly. Over the years there have been many discussions about the classification of diabetes and none is entirely satisfactory.

Management

Factors to be considered

- The patient's and the doctor's educational and general background
- The patient's and the doctor's previous encounters with diabetes
- The patient's current mental and physical state
- The type of diabetes and its treatment
- The situation (e.g. in a surgery, clinic, patient's home)
- Other support available for the patient (e.g. family, friends)
- Other professional support (e.g. diabetes specialist nurses)

What is wrong with me, doctor?

Most doctors and nurses are so familiar with medical terminology, anatomy, physiology, and biochemistry that it can be difficult remembering what it was like not knowing where organs and systems are and how they work. Furthermore, many people are unused to processing information in a logical way. Remember that patients may forget verbal information. Give them a booklet or tape to take home. There are several books which could be recommended (p. 222).

Tell the patient he or she has diabetes and that this means that there is too much sugar in the blood.

The other essential facts are that this is a lifelong condition which will always need regular checks by the patient and the diabetes team. It will not disappear but it can be controlled by careful attention to diet and, if necessary, to medication. (Never talk about 'mild' diabetes—this is grievously misleading—diabetes controlled by diet alone can still maim or blind.) Ensure that the person realizes that diabetes rarely interferes with work, home life, or activities and that it is compatible with keeping fit. Be positive. Explain that with careful attention to management, the risk of further health damage from diabetes can be minimized.

Give the patient time to ask questions or express worries.

What is diabetes?

There are two main facets to cover:

1 The concept of glucose imbalance and the role of the pancreas and insulin; and
2 Diabetes as a disorder which can affect the whole body over the years.

The patient should know that in diabetes the body is unable to use glucose (or sugar) as a fuel and that because glucose cannot be taken up by the body tissues, it builds up in the bloodstream. Eventually, the glucose overflows into the urine making it thick and syrupy which draws water out of the body producing large amounts of urine and causing thirst. Patients who require insulin need to know about the pancreas and its failure to produce insulin. Although one does not wish to frighten people who have newly diagnosed diabetes it is important that they realize that diabetes is not just sugar trouble. The concept of diabetes as a multisystem disorder should be introduced at the outset and gently amplified over subsequent sessions.

Why me?

Although the diabetes team may be more interested in assessing and treating the patient, the person with diabetes has a strong need to know why they have the condition. Failure to address this may hold up the patient's acceptance of his or her condition and learning about self care. There may be a strong family history and a few patients will have drug-induced diabetes or other hormone conditions.

What next?

Start treatment promptly:

◆ a simple diet

◆ self-monitoring

◆ basic diabetes education

◆ for some patients: insulin or oral hypoglycaemic drugs.

Each of these aspects is dealt with more fully in subsequent chapters.

Diet

Is the patient fat or thin? If fat they need to eat less of everything, especially fat and sugar. If thin they can eat what their appetite dictates.

Encourage starchy carbohydrates with plenty of fibre (for example, pulses, wholemeal foods). Encourage vegetables with fruit in moderation. Discourage sugar, sweet foods, and soft drinks; discourage fatty foods.

If the patient has Type 2 diabetes but does not have severe symptoms they should initially try adjusting their diet, whatever their blood glucose level. Do not give potent glucose-lowering drugs to patients who could manage on diet alone.

> Mrs Bibi was referred to the Diabetic clinic. Her diabetes was diagnosed four weeks previously at a well-person clinic and had been confirmed by a random blood glucose of 11.5 mmol/l and a fasting glucose of 8.0 mmol/l. She complained of weakness but when pressed for details seemed unable to give a clear history. Her daughter said the family had cut out all sugar from her diet and restricted the portions of food at all meals. She had been taking her tablets every day as instructed. The tablets were glibenclamide, 5 mg daily. The patient seemed vague and was unsteady on her feet. Her daughter confirmed that her mother had seemed confused at home for the past three weeks. A clinic glucose measurement was 1.4 mmol/l. She was admitted and her glucose was restored to normal. Subsequently her blood glucose was normal on diet alone.

Glucose-lowering medication

It may be difficult to decide which treatment to give to whom. While there are some rules, there is undoubtedly a grey area in which the treatment decision is a blend of experience and trial and error. If someone is insulin deficient he or she needs insulin. If someone has an additional acute major illness, especially infection, he or she usually needs insulin.

If there is no evidence of major tissue breakdown or major infection, especially if the person is of an age and habit suggesting Type 2 diabetes, the treatment is diet for all patients and oral hypoglycaemic therapy for many. These options will succeed only if the patient is making insulin.

Many people with newly diagnosed diabetes are convinced that they will need regular injections: this may be a terrifying thought. As soon as it has become apparent that the patient does not need insulin, they should be told. Otherwise the patient may be so worried about the prospect of 'the needle' that everything else you say will be forgotten. In many cases the treatment decision can be made in the first few minutes of a consultation.

Insulin

People who usually need insulin have most of the following characteristics:

◆ under 40 years old

◆ thin

◆ severe diabetic symptoms

◆ marked weight loss

◆ profuse urinary ketones

◆ serious infection

◆ another major acute illness

Insulin treatment should be started within 24 hours of diagnosis, preferably immediately. It is vital that the diabetes specialist nurse or other teacher has sufficient protected time to teach the patient the necessary skills. If possible the patient should give the first injection. Otherwise a subcutaneous injection of 4–10 units of soluble insulin (for example Actrapid, Humulin S) can be given immediately, and the diabetes specialist nurse can visit the patient at home or see him/her separately to teach the technique (p. 82).

Insulin regimens are discussed in detail in Chapter 9. A simple starting regimen to use at home is a fixed proportion mixture such as Mixtard 30 g.e., Mixtard 30 pen, or Humulin M3, giving 4–10 units s.c. twice daily. The disposable pre-loaded pens containing Mixtard 30 are easiest for most new patients.

Oral hypoglycaemic drugs

The use of oral hypoglycaemic drugs is discussed more fully in Chapter 8. People who usually need oral hypoglycaemics have the following characteristics:

◆ Do not need insulin.

◆ Plasma glucose over 6 mmol/l fasting or over 8 mmol/l random despite a diabetic diet (some people are already eating a diet similar to that advised for people with diabetes).

◆ Marked symptoms (these may settle rapidly on diet alone but some physicians would prescribe oral hypoglycaemic drugs for rapid symptom relief and then reduce the dose as dietary measures take effect. Careful monitoring is needed to avoid hypoglycaemia).

As much care should be taken to educate patients about their tablets as is taken with insulin injections. They are not a cure for diabetes and do not mean that the person has 'mild' diabetes (there is no such thing). They work only while he or she is making insulin. If insulin production fails (and this often happens over the years) the patient will need insulin injections. Tablets cannot work properly if the patient does not stick to his diet. They are a long-term treatment and not just a week's course.

WARNINGS

The following warnings are essential for patients newly started on glucose-lowering medication

- Hypoglycaemia—know what it is, how to recognize it, how to treat it.
- Do not drive or operate machinery or perform other potentially hazardous activities for one week (adjust according to situation).
- Carry diabetes card.
- Carry glucose.

Self-monitoring

This is as important as medication. It allows both the patient and diabetes team to monitor the response to treatment and to the patient's eating and activity (Chapters 6 and 7). Blood testing is best but urine testing is adequate for Type 2 patients in whom a lack of glucose in post-prandial urine samples has been confirmed to be associated with normal or near-normal glycosylated haemoglobin levels. It is essential to teach the technique properly at the outset, otherwise it is a waste of time and blood or urine.

Initially, patients should check their blood glucose before each meal and before bed. Once the blood glucose has returned towards normal, people with Type 2 diabetes can reduce the frequency, the fasting blood glucose (or postprandial urine glucose) being the most useful measurement.

Driving

Warn patients on glucose-lowering treatment about the risk of hypoglycaemia. People with diabetes should inform the licensing authority (DVLA, Swansea) of their condition. They must also inform their motor insurance company.

Help

The patient should leave clutching the telephone number of a diabetes adviser (this may be the general practitioner, the practice nurse, if trained in diabetes care, or a diabetes specialist nurse) whom they can contact if they have any further queries.

Give the patient clear instructions to telephone if help is needed. He or she will also need to know whom to contact for supplies.

Finally, give the patient written instructions about the next appointment.

Summary

- If you are not trained in diabetes care, someone who is should assess the person with newly diagnosed diabetes. Patients aged under 20 years should always be managed by a specialist diabetes service.
- Do not delay treatment of clinically ill patients. Telephone your local diabetologist or acute medical on-take team immediately.
- Problems requiring urgent hospital assessment and probably admission include: impaired conscious level, vomiting, hyperventilation, severe dehydration, low blood pressure, fever, foot or leg infection or gangrene, blood glucose over 25 mmol/l, concomitant severe illness, especially infection.
- Insulin treatment is also needed for severe symptoms, profuse urinary ketones, marked weight loss, and 90 per cent of those under 30 years of age.
- Referral letters should include the diagnostic glucose levels.
- All people with newly diagnosed diabetes should be fully assessed by detailed history and clinical examination.
- Perform baseline investigations.
- Tell the patient he or she has diabetes, what it is, and why. Discuss the management plan with them. Give them take-home information.
- Initial management should be simple—diet, glucose-lowering medication if neeeded, and self-glucose monitoring.
- Warn of hypoglycaemia when prescribing glucose-lowering drugs. These patients must carry glucose and a diabetic card.
- Warn drivers about hypoglycaemia. They must also inform the DVLA and their insurance company of their diabetes.
- Tell the patient how to get help.
- Give the patient his or her next appointment.

Chapter 3

The aims of diabetes care

To enjoy life to the full

The aim should be for a person with diabetes to enjoy life to the full without their diabetes or its care causing problems now or in the future.

Many people with diabetes simply want to 'get back to normal'. Although this is a term used frequently in everyday speech, normality is hard to define. Dictionary definitions for normal include 'ordinary', 'well-adjusted', 'functioning regularly'. Each person will have their own personal definition. It is devastating to discover that one has a permanent illness which may disable or kill you, which requires uncomfortable and sometimes complex treatment, and which may impact on one's job, driving, insurance, and family life. It is misleading and unfair to paint too rosy a picture of life with diabetes but neither should carers paint too gloomy a future. Help people with diabetes to get back towards their version of normal as soon as possible. If this is not feasible then provide them with sympathetic and practical support through their disappointment and frustration. Help them to build a new 'normality'.

Diabetes education (see also Chapter 4)

People with diabetes need to understand what diabetes is, what it means for them personally and what may happen in the future. They need to learn what they themselves can do to reduce the likelihood of glucose problems and tissue complications, and what their diabetes team can do to help them. They should understand how best to use their medication and related technology, how to cope with common difficulties and emergencies, how to seek help, and how to make the most of health resources. Relatives and friends also want to learn and help.

Education is a continuous process so there must be opportunities for learning during every interaction with health care staff—and in between. People need revision sessions and opportunities to extend and update their knowledge.

Appropriate, accessible, high-standard, evidence-based health care

Each person with diabetes should be able to access diabetes care when and where they need it, easily and without barriers. Distant surgeries or clinics, too few diabetes-trained staff, poor public transport, over-busy tired staff, lack of continuity of staff, and lack of expert advice out-of-hours are some examples of barriers to care. Some can be resolved by increasing resources, some by additional training.

Staff delivering diabetes care should know about diabetes. Obvious? Apparently not. Many patients are cared for by health care staff who have had no special training in diabetes care. Nowadays this is not acceptable. Over the past 10 years the publication of several large, well-planned studies has provided a clear, evidence-based blue-print for diabetes care (see p. 33). All those caring for diabetic patients should follow this to the best of their ability. They should update themselves as new evidence emerges. The problem for health care staff working in the NHS is that the resources to do what we know we need to do are not always available, especially as the frequency of diabetes increases. This means we must use what we have efficiently, with good communication within and between primary and secondary care, and no duplication or omission. Staff should be supported with good training, updating, and good working conditions.

Each patient is unique

Daisy lives alone since her husband died. She is 81, walks with a stick, and is blind in one eye. She has peripheral vascular disease and arthritis and has had several falls. She takes gliclazide for her Type 2 diabetes. Her blood pressure is 165/95 and her HbA1$_c$ is 8.3% (normal range 4.5–6.5% for that laboratory).

Malcolm is a successful 32-year-old businessman. He has had diabetes for five years treated with gliclazide. He works long hours and regards his job as stressful. He enjoys playing football at weekends. His blood pressure is 165/95 and his HbA1$_c$ is 8.3% (normal range 4.5–6.5%).

Clearly these two patients are very different. One is elderly and frail, the other young and energetic. One has plenty of time for herself, the other is in a stressful, time-consuming job. One finds finger-prick glucose measurements difficult, the other easy. One does not drive and cannot use a bus, the other has a car. Both have elevated blood pressures and poor glucose balance. So what factors influence the targets we set for Daisy and Malcolm?

If it doesn't work for me, it doesn't work

The care plan we produce must be acceptable to the patient and they must feel that it will work for them. As with all patients we need to consider their previous knowledge of their condition and its care, their attitudes, their expectations, their emotional state, their educational level, and factors which may impede understanding. Primary care staff are often thought to be better at this than those in secondary care. They usually know the patient and their circumstances better. They often know relatives who may have a considerable bearing on the patient's behaviour.

Physical factors

Factors affecting understanding (e.g. dementia, metabolic disarray), movement and mobility (arthritis, stroke, amputation), sensation (neuropathy), balance (stroke, postural hypotension), concentration (malaise from persistent hyperglycaemia, pain), vision (cataract, retinopathy), and hearing (diabetic deafness) can all impede care.

One does not aim for a blood pressure of 125/75 in someone with postural hypotension, for example.

Practicalities

Modern diabetes care means that the patient must be reviewed more often. He or she needs to be able to get to the surgery or clinic easily. If not, the care should go to them. We should also consider making better use of the telephone and e-mail (with appropriate confidentiality). In Hillingdon, NHS Direct and the Local Diabetes Services Advisory Group have pioneered the Hillingdon Diabetes Support Network— a helpline run by NHS Direct using nurses trained in diabetes care. In other areas there have long been excellent specialist helplines. However, it is often those patients who have most difficulties hearing or using the phone who cannot get to the surgery.

It is easier to look after your diabetes if you are financially well off. Meters are not yet available on the NHS so have to be bought. It is easier to enjoy an attractive diabetic diet if you can afford interesting food. So we must ensure that low-income patients can access good care. Now that we are encouraging more frequent check-ups, patients may be worried that they may lose their jobs, those with young families may find it hard to find babysitters, and students may miss school or college. Late evening or weekend surgeries are valued by patients but have to be staffed.

NHS care arrangements are complicated, especially if you have a disability such as amputation, and the planned links between health and social care are welcome. Diabetic patients are often under the care of multiple medical teams. Daisy, for example, sees her GP, the diabetic clinic, the eye clinic, the vascular clinic, the rheumatologist, the orthopaedic clinic. She has an appointment for care of the elderly about her falls. She sees a chiropodist separately, has a social worker, and her son recently arranged a visit to an osteopath.

Evidence-based diabetes care for adults

There can be few chronic disorders which offer so much scope for preventive health care as diabetes. This section discusses the practical application of some recent, large studies of diabetes care or subset analyses of studies including diabetic patients. Study acronyms are given, and references and useful reading are on p. 33.

There is now clear evidence that good diabetes care reduces diabetic tissue damage. In the past, it was usual to produce targets which indicated 'perfect, acceptable, and unacceptable' diabetes care. We must aim for perfect diabetes care for all, tailoring our final decision to take account of the patient's situation and wishes. Clearly, we must not endanger patients in our search for the perfect glucose or perfect blood pressure. At the same time, studies have demonstrated that, with care, one can achieve considerable improvements in both without major physical or emotional side-effects. The world of research studies, with frequent discussions with research nurses or doctors, is very different from the busy surgery with too many patients and too few staff. The resourcing of modern diabetes care is a national issue. In the meantime we need to focus on the key care issues for our patients and try to deliver them as efficiently and kindly as possible.

The targets

The aim of diabetes care is to return the patient to as close a non-diabetic state as is safe and practical for that particular person. The targets are set out in Appendix A. Please note that they apply to adults. Children also need careful diabetes care, aiming for safe, near normalization of parameters, but this has particular risks in children. They should be cared for by specialist teams. I have deliberately chosen the most stringent targets available from current literature, recognizing that they will not be possible in some patients and that care is needed in their application. There is increasing evidence that there is no threshold effect for blood pressure or glucose providing they remain within physiological levels (i.e. providing adequate perfusion and cerebral glucose delivery respectively). There appears to be no threshold effect for cholesterol either, although research continues. Risk reduction will also be discussed in the chapters on complications of diabetes.

Stop smoking!

People with diabetes who smoke have at least the same risk of morbidity and mortality as non-diabetics who smoke, and probably greater. Diabetics who smoke have about four times the risk of dying from a cardiovascular disease as those who do not. Vigorous efforts should be made to discourage young people with diabetes from starting smoking. Smokers should be given considerable help and support to stop. As nicotine may alter the rate of insulin absorption, glucose should be monitored after stopping. The insulin dose may need to be adjusted. Nicotine patches can be used by people with diabetes but care should be taken by those with cardiovascular disease. Avoid patches in those with renal failure. Bupropion can also be used in people with diabetes but not in those with renal failure. Monitor blood pressure.

Blood pressure control (see also Chapter 13)

Good blood pressure control is more important than good glucose control in reducing cardiovascular disease although both matter. Cardiovascular disease is the commonest cause of death in diabetic patients. There is substantial evidence that reducing blood pressure greatly reduces the risk of diabetic and cardiovascular events—fatal and non-fatal. In UKPDS (38) tight blood pressure control produced a mean blood pressure of 144/82 mm Hg compared with the less tight control group's 154/87 mm Hg. The tight control group showed a 24 per cent reduction in diabetes-related endpoints, with a 32 per cent reduction in deaths due to diabetes, 44 per cent reduction in strokes and 37 per cent reduction in microvascular endpoints.

Advice about blood pressure targets varies. Diabetes UK and the National Institute of Clinical Excellence (NICE) (2002) state that the blood pressure should be below 140/80 (below 135/75 in people with renal disease). The Joint British Societies (2000) advocated a blood pressure at rest below 130/80, and below 125/75 in someone with any degree of renal impairment. Lower targets are likely to achieve greater protection from tissue damage, providing postural hypotension can be avoided. A lot of patients with diabetes need treatment. See Appendix A.

Angiotensin-converting enzyme (ACE) inhibitors (captopril (UKPDS), enalapril (ABCD), fosinopril (FACET, HOT), ramipril (HOPE, MICRO-HOPE), beta blockers (atenolol (UKPDS)) and diuretic agents (bendrofluazide (UKPDS), hydrochloro-thiazide (Syst-EUR)) are all effective and do not produce adverse metabolic effects in diabetic patients. They are usually used in combination. Calcium channel blockers have shown variable results—felodipine (HOT) and nitrendipine (Syst-EUR) were safe and effective; further research is awaited.

The risk is of hypotension—sustained or postural. Postural hypotension is particu-larly likely in the elderly and in people with autonomic neuropathy and it should be remembered that most people with peripheral neuropathy will have a degree of auto-nomic neuropathy. Ask patients about dizziness on standing. It is obviously helpful to measure lying and standing blood pressure, but even if there is no drop patients may still have postural symptoms at other times. Give medication at night if possible. It is usually possible to find a treatment regimen which achieves the target blood pressure without postural hypotension—combination therapy is often more successful than large doses of a single agent. The commonest cause of failure to reach the desired target is failure to take the tablets.

The use of atenolol and captopril did not increase hypoglycaemia in Type 2 diabetes (UKPDS). However, patients on insulin should be warned that beta blockers may reduce their warning of hypoglycaemia. Patients with poor warning of hypoglycaemia should avoid beta blockers.

Blood glucose control (see also Chapters 7–11)

Intensive blood glucose control reduces the development and progression of the complications of diabetes (DCCT, UKPDS). In DCCT, the intensively-treated group of Type 1 diabetic patients had a mean blood glucose concentration of 8.6 mmol/l compared with 12.8 mmol/l in the conventionally treated group. Intensive therapy reduced the risk of developing new retinopathy by 76 per cent, and, in those with pre-existing retinopathy, slowed its progression by 54 per cent. Overall, intensive therapy reduced occurrence of microalbuminuria by 39 per cent, overt proteinuria by 54 per cent, and clinical neuropathy by 54 per cent. In UKPDS (34), intensive treatment with metformin in overweight Type 2 patients produced a median $HbA1_c$ of 7.4 per cent compared with 8.0 per cent in those treated conventionally. Intensive treatment with metformin reduced any diabetes-related endpoint by 32 per cent. In UKPDS (33), intensive treatment of Type 2 patients with sulphonylurea or insulin reduced $HbA1_c$ to 7.0 per cent compared with 7.9 per cent with conventional treatment. This reduced any diabetes endpoint by 12 per cent.

Intensive blood glucose control increased the frequency of hypoglycaemia, espe-cially in Type 1 diabetes, but careful attention to blood glucose monitoring, good access to knowledgeable advice, and appropriate treatment adjustment can reduce this. One obvious question is whether quality of life was impaired by all these finger-pricks, frequent clinic attendances, the risk of hypoglycaemia, and so on. Quality of life was no different between intensively and conventionally treated patients. Intensive glucose lowering did not appear to have an adverse effect upon cognitive function.

The closer the HbA1$_c$ is to the non-diabetic range, the lower the risk of diabetic tissue damage. Thus the aim for blood glucose is that observed in non-diabetics and those without any glucose intolerance. This means a fasting blood glucose between 4 and 6 mmol/l. At other times the glucose should be between 4 and 8 mmol/l. The HbA1$_c$ should be within the normal range for your local laboratory. For detailed discussion of glucose-lowering agents see Chapters 8 and 9.

The main risk is of hypoglycaemia (see Chapter 10). Every patient on glucose-lowering treatment (whether tablets or insulin) must be taught how to recognize and treat hypoglycaemia. They should also know how to adjust their treatment to reduce the risk of further hypoglycaemia. Patients with varied timetables, varied meals, and varied exercise and those who have problems being careful with their diabetes are particularly at risk of hypoglycaemia, as are the very young and elderly. Any patient who has had one hypoglycaemic attack is likely to have more. Some patients will be unable to achieve a normal glucose without hypoglycaemia. In this case you must work together towards the best compromise between safety now and good health long term.

Lipid lowering (see also Chapter 13)

Good glucose control also reduces lipids (DCCT, UKPDS). A low-fat, high-fibre, weight-normalizing diet also reduces lipids if rigorously adhered to. However, many patients find this difficult and one should not wait more than a few months to see if dietary efforts have reduced lipids before considering medication. Check for other causes of hyperlipidaemia.

The Heart Protection Study (HPS) included 20 536 patients aged 40 to 80 years at high risk of coronary disease but who did not fulfil existing criteria for cholesterol-lowering therapy in 1994. They included many subjects with diabetes. Preliminary results show that after five years of simvastatin treatment (40 mg daily) 2831 patients had died—1328 out of 10 269 (12.9 per cent) on simvastatin vs. 1503 out of 10 267 (14.6 per cent) on placebo ($2p<0.001$); 19.9 per cent of patients had a vascular event on simvastatin compared with 25.4 per cent on placebo. Simvastatin prevented major cardiac and other vascular events in 70 of every 1000 diabetic participants over 40 years old when compared with those on placebo. HPS also showed that simvastatin is safe—there was no significant difference in elevation of liver enzyme or of muscle enzyme between the two groups. (Preliminary communication, American Heart Association meeting 2001; *www.hpsinfo.org*).

In subgroup analysis of other studies, statins (lovastatin (AFCAPS/TexCAPS)) and fibrates (gemfibrozil (Helsinki), bezafibrate (SENDCAP)) reduced myocardial infarcts and/or cardiac death in diabetic patients. In studies of patients after myocardial infarction, statins (simvastatin (4S), pravastatin (CARE, LIPID)) reduced cardiac events and death. In DAIS (731), diabetic patients with coronary artery disease (half without previously known cardiac disease) and mild lipoprotein abnormalities were given micronized fenofibrate or placebo. Those on fenofibrate had slower narrowing of their coronary artery lesions than those on placebo.

There are two ways of producing targets for lipid lowering. One is to look at a chart such as the Joint British Societies Coronary Risk Prediction Chart which uses the ratio of total: HDL cholesterol and other risk factors to identify 10 years' risk of coronary heart disease (Joint British Societies 2000). The other is to set a cut-off for lipid levels. The danger of introducing complex charts to plan treatment is that some staff may feel 'I am too busy to fiddle around with sums' and simply use guesswork—or do nothing. Furthermore, one needs to read the small print to correct for family history and so on. Simpler targets are more likely to be used. The Joint British Societies recommendation for people with diabetes is a total cholesterol below 5 mmol/l. LDL cholesterol should be below 3 mmol/l. However, the findings of HPS imply that using these thresholds is inappropriate—many of the patients included had falls of cholesterol well below these levels.

Fasting triglycerides should be below 2.3 mmol, and some say below 1.5 mmol/l (ensure that the patient has fasted). Note that elevated triglyceride and reduced HDL cholesterol also increase the risk of cardiovascular disease. For triglyceride levels over 2.3 mmol/l, institute rigorous blood glucose control and reduction of alcohol intake. If the triglyceride is between 2.3 and 5 mmol/l use atorvastatin or 80 mg doses of simvastatin. Triglyceride levels above 5 mmol/l are unlikely to respond to a statin and a fibrate should be used. Monitor liver function with both statins and fibrates.

Bearing in mind the very high risk of coronary artery disease in diabetes and the possible plaque stabilizing role of statins, in addition to lipid lowering, one should consider early initiation of drug treatment See Appendix A. Use a statin for patients with a cholesterol over 5 mmol/l and a triglyceride below 5.0 mmol/l. (The triglyceride level is arbitrary and based on practical experience.)

Normalize weight

Obesity increases insulin resistance, blood pressure, and cardiovascular risk. Weight reduction reduces symptoms of diabetes and reduces the treatment needed to normalize blood glucose levels. It is therefore worthwhile encouraging weight loss in people with diabetes (Douketis 1999). The aim is a body mass index (BMI) between 18 and 25 kg/m^2. In general, the most effective weight reduction strategy combines dietary advice (see Chapter 5), regular exercise (see Chapter 12), and long-term help in changing everyday weight-gaining habits. Very low-calorie diets are successful. So is orlistat, which inhibits pancreatic lipase and therefore induces fat malabsorption (and frequent gastrointestinal side-effects). However, both require expert supervision and long-term dietetic support.

Identification and treatment of tissue damage

While the main thrust of diabetes care must be prevention of problems, the sad reality is that over a third of patients with Type 2 diabetes have obvious tissue damage at the time of diagnosis. There is evidence from Diabetes UK's audit data and regression calculations that the onset of coronary heart disease culminating in myocardial infarction is 20 years pre-diagnosis; stroke, 12 years; nephropathy, 18 years; amputation, 7 years; and retinopathy, 7 years (see p. 5). At least half the patients with diabetes on any practice list will have overt tissue damage. Every person with diabetes must be assumed to have hidden tissue damage.

Many diabetic complications have specific treatments and their progress can be slowed by redoubled preventive care (see above and Chapters 12 and 13). It is therefore essential to detect any hint of tissue damage early. This means rigorous checks by the patient (reporting visual change, foot problems, etc.) and by health care professionals. Standards for monitoring are described in the relevant chapters. Negative information (e.g. normal foot pulses, no retinopathy) must be recorded as well as positive findings. Tissue damage is checked annually at present, although there is no evidence to support a 12-month interval as being better than a shorter or longer one. In a perfect world we should probably check more often. The patient questionnaire used in the Hillingdon Consensus Care Project (see Appendix A) is one attempt to introduce more frequent, structured checks on warning symptoms in a time-efficient way. But the main difficulty lies in the latency of much severe tissue damage until it is too late to prevent disability.

Diabetes register; audit and recall system

In order to deliver good diabetes care each unit or practice needs to know who has diabetes in their area of responsibility and what care they have had. This means a register with audit facilities. There should be a recall system for annual review and, optimally, reminders for interim check-ups. Non-attenders have a high rate of complications and should be pursued in a constructive way.

Local support

There should be a local forum for supporting district-wide diabetes care. In many districts this is the Local Diabetes Services Advisory Group. There should be representation from all those involved in receiving, providing, and purchasing diabetes care throughout the district. Such a group can be a major force in communication, education, and improving resources.

Cost-effectiveness

Many health service financial cycles are annual. Diabetic complications take years to become obvious, so the immediate benefits of intensive management can rarely be demonstrated to a financial manager planning the following year's budget. Both DCCT and UKPDS studied the long-term cost-effectiveness of intensive diabetes care. In UKPDS, intensive management of Type 2 diabetic patients 'significantly increased treatment costs but substantially reduced the cost of complications and increased the time free from complications'. They calculated that with intensive care the patient would gain 1.14 years (confidence interval 0.69–1.61) of event-free time (an event being a diabetic complication, including death). They did not include the nonmedical and social benefits such as fitness to work. In DCCT, they concluded that intensive rather than conventional therapy for the 120 000 people with Type 1 diabetes in the

United States would gain 920 000 years of sight, 691 000 years free from end-stage renal disease, 678 000 years free from lower extremity amputation, and 611 000 years of life.

References and further reading

ABCD Estacio, R.O., Jeffers, B.W., Hiatt, W.R., *et al.* (1998). The effect of nisoldipine as compared with enalapril on cardiovascular events in patients with non-insulin dependent diabetes and hypertension. *N Eng J Med*, **338**, 645–52.

AFCAPS/TexCAPS Downs, J.R., Clearfield, M., Weis, S., *et al.* (1998). Primary prevention of acute coronary events with lovastatin in men and women with average cholesterol levels; results of AFCAPS/TexCAPS. Air Force/Texas Coronary Atherosclerosis Prevention Study. *JAMA*, **279**, 1615–22.

CARE Sacks, F.M., Pfeffer, M.A., Moye, L.A., *et al.* (1996). The effect of pravastatin on coronary events after myocardial infarction in patients with average cholesterol levels. Cholesterol and Recurrent Events Trial investigators. *N Engl J Med*, **335**(14), 1001–9.

DAIS Diabetes Atherosclerosis Intervention Study Investigators (2001). Effect of fenofibrate on progression of coronary-artery disease in type 2 diabetes: the Diabetes Atherosclerosis Intervention Study, a randomised study. *Lancet*, **357**, 905–10.

DCCT

DCCT Research Group (1993). The effect of intensive treatment of diabetes on the development and progression of long-term complications in insulin-dependent diabetes mellitus. *N Engl J Med*, **329**(14), 977–86.

DCCT Research Group (1995). Effect of intensive diabetes management on macrovascular events and risk factors in the Diabetes Control and Complications Trial. *Am J Cardiol*, **75**, 894–903.

DCCT Research Group (1996). Lifetime benefits and costs of intensive therapy as practiced in the Diabetes Control and Complications Trial. *JAMA*, **276**, 1409–15.

Douketis, J.D., Feightner, J.W., Attia, J., *et al.* (1999). Periodic health examination, 1999 update: 1. Detection, prevention and treatment of obesity. Canadian Task Force on Preventive Health Care. *CMAJ*, **160**, 513–25.

FACET Tatti, P., Pahor, M., Byington, R.P., *et al.* (1998). Outcome results of the Fosinopril versus Amlodipine Cardiovascular Events randomised Trial (FACET) in patients with hypertension and NIDDM. *Diabetes Care*, **21**, 597–603.

Helsinki Koskinen, P., Manttari, M., Manninen, V., *et al.* (1992). Coronary heart disease incidence in NIDDM patients in the Helsinki Heart Study. *Diabetes Care*, **15**, 820–5.

HOPE/MICRO-HOPE Heart Outcomes Prevention Evaluation (HOPE) Study Investigators (2000). Effects of ramipril on cardiovascular and microvascular outcomes in people with diabetes mellitus; results of the HOPE and MICRO-HOPE sub study. *Lancet*, **355**, 253–9.

HOT Hansson, L., Zanchetti, A., Carruthers, S.G., *et al.* (1998). Effects of intensive blood pressure lowering and low-dose aspirin in patients with hypertension; principal results of the Hypertension Optimal Treatment (HOT) randomised trial. *Lancet* **351**, 1755–62.

Joint British Societies British Cardiac Society, British Hyperlipidaemia Association, British Hypertension Society, British Diabetic Association (2000). Joint British recommendations on prevention of coronary heart disease in clinical practice: summary. *BMJ*, **320**, 705–8.

LIPID The Long-term Intervention with Pravastatin In Ischemic Disease (LIPID) Study Program (1998). Prevention of cardiovascular events and death with pravastatin in patients with coronary heart disease and a broad range of initial cholesterol levels. *N Engl J Med*, **339**, 1349–57.

NICE (National Institute for Clinical Excellence)

NICE (2002). Management of Type 2 diabetes. Renal disease—prevention and early management. Inherited Clinical Guideline F. *www.nice.org.uk*

NICE (2002). Management of Type 2 diabetes. Retinopathy—screening and early management. Inherited Clinical Guideline E. *www.nice.org.uk*

SENDCAP Elkeles, R.S., Diamond, J.R., Poulter, C., *et al.* (1998). Cardiovascular outcomes in Type 2 diabetes. A double-blind, placebo controlled study of bezafibrate; the St Mary's, Ealing, Northwick Park Diabetes Cardiovascular Prevention (SENDCAP) Study. *Diabetes Care*, **21**, 641–8.

4S Pyorala, K., Pedersen, T.R., Kjekshus, J. *et al.* (1997). Cholesterol lowering with simvastatin improves prognosis of diabetic patients with coronary heart disease. A subgroup analysis of the Scandinavian Simvastatin Survival Study. *Diabetes Care*, **20**, 614–20.

Syst-EUR Staessen, J.A., Fagard, R., Thijs, L. *et al.* (1998). Subgroup and per-protocol analysis of the randomized European Trial on Isolated Systolic Hypertension in the Elderly. *Arch Int Med*, **158**, 1681–91.

UKPDS (UK Prospective Diabetes Study Group)

UKPDS (1998). Intensive blood-glucose control with sulphonylureas or insulin compared with conventional treatment and risk of complications in patients with type 2 diabetes. (UKPDS 33). *Lancet* **352**, 837–53.

UKPDS (1998). Effect of intensive blood-glucose control with metformin on complications of overweight patients with type 2 diabetes. (UKPDS 34). *Lancet*, **352**, 854–65.

UKPDS (1998). Tight blood pressure control and risk of macrovascular and microvascular complications in type 2 diabetes. (UKPDS 38). *BMJ*, **317**, 703–13.

UKPDS (1998). Efficacy of atenolol and captopril in reducing risk of macrovascular and microvascular complications in type 2 diabetes. (UKPDS 39) *BMJ*, **317**, 713–20.

Gray, A., Raikou, M., McGuire, A., *et al.*, on behalf of the UKPDS (2000). Cost effectiveness of an intensive blood glucose control policy in patients with type 2 diabetes: economic analysis alongside randomised controlled trial. (UKPDS 41). *BMJ*, **320**, 1373–8.

Chapter 4

Diabetes education

Diabetes education is essential to patient survival. If you have appendicitis, you go to hospital and the surgeon removes the inflamed appendix. All the patient has to do is lie there whilst the operation is performed. Afterwards some effort is required to start eating again and to mobilize—but the doctors and nurses tell you what to do. In other words, the patient presents the professionals with the problem and they take it away. This process requires little health care knowledge by the patient other than the realization that if your tummy hurts a lot it is a good idea to call a doctor. (Of course, the patient may have a less frightening time if the professionals do explain fully.)

Diabetes is very different. It is a chronic lifelong disorder. More importantly, it is the person who has the condition who determines the outcome. The professionals provide advice and a management plan. It is up to the patient to follow this on a day-to-day basis and to expand and adapt it to their particular circumstances. Problems may arise which require a logical extension of the instructions given by the doctor or nurse. The situation may deteriorate and the patient has to know when to seek help, and how urgently.

Ask if the patient has a close relative or friend with whom they wish to share the teaching session. Often relatives are more worried about the diabetes than the person who has it. They may harbour misconceptions which subsequently override what you have said. They can also reinforce the diabetes teaching and correct patients' misconceptions. Being allowed to share in the diabetes experience can help relatives overcome feelings of uselessness. 'I want to help but I don't know what to do.'

There are two agendas in any teaching session. The teacher's—what should be taught, and the learner's—what I want to learn. These are rarely identical. If a professional does not address the patient's agenda, the information given in the lesson may be ignored or at best half-remembered. It is easy to launch into a standard lesson: what is diabetes, what is hypoglycaemia, etc. but it may be better to find out what the patient wants to know first. 'No question is ever stupid if it has to be a question' (Thomas, personal communication).

Many people do not know how their body works. Breathing, circulation, digestion are all mysterious. Patients may have startling misconceptions, for example that babies emerge through the umbilicus, or that the gall-bladder drains bile into the blood (this one has been around for hundreds of years). The basic knowledge required to understand about diabetes is rarely complete. Few lay people know how food is digested and how the products of digestion are converted into energy. Few can indicate where the pancreas is, and what it does. Even people who should have good understanding of human physiology and anatomy may harbour gross misconceptions—a woman stumbled into a diabetic clinic in tears having been informed by a midwife that she had miscarried because she was injecting her insulin into the subcutaneous tissue of her abdomen. Another woman, newly diagnosed with diabetes said, 'I knew three things about diabetes—you lose your legs, your eyes, and your mind'. Diabetes is usually linked with sugar in the public mind but people are not always sure whether it is too much or too little sugar that is the problem. It is often linked with needles and coma too.

One cannot start a teaching session without making some assessment of the patient's general characteristics and level of health knowledge. Who is the person? What do they already know? What are their thoughts and attitudes? Who else influences them? The patient's motivation is crucial. Adult learning is usually most enthusiastic when related to solving problems and aiming for specific, not-too-distant, goals. They have lost some of the childhood joys of discovery. In general, use of the 'teachable moment'— the time when the person formulates the question or needs to know how to resolve a problem—engenders more interest and may lead to better retention of knowledge. However, while one can utilize those teachable moments which occur in front of professionals, one cannot wait until they happen. Some more formalized teaching is needed.

What does the patient want to know?

'Is it serious?' 'Am I going to die?' 'Will I get better?' 'Am I going to lose my legs like that lady in the waiting room?' 'Will I go blind?' 'Will I lose my job?' 'Am I going to lose my driving licence?' 'Will I lose my boyfriend?' 'What are you going to do to me now?' 'Will I need to have injections?' 'Will it hurt?' These are among the questions in most peoples' minds when they discover that they are ill. 'What is diabetes?' may be further down the patient's list than one expects. Once the shock of diagnosis is over other questions relating to living with diabetes emerge—what diabetes is, what it means, what diet and other treatment are needed, how to use the appropriate technology (e.g. finger-prick blood glucose testing, needles, syringes), selfcare, the prevention of short-term and long-term complications, and how to care for diabetes under different circumstances. Practicalities such as clinic/surgery arrangements and whom to call for help also need to be covered.

Unlike school teachers, doctors have no formal teacher training, although there are now some opportunities for such, for example the Primary Diabetes Course at the University of Warwick. Increasingly diabetes specialist nurses do attend workshops and courses in this field. But most have to learn by doing. Some common sense ideas may help.

One can teach anywhere but it is easier if the teacher and patient(s) sit in a quiet, undisturbed place with sufficient time for full explanations. This rules out most diabetic clinics, although the clinic set-up could be changed. The teacher should be able to give the student his undivided attention—no telephone calls or bleeps. People are more likely to remember things if they are involved in the lesson—discussion or question-and-answer format rather than lecture. Use visual aids—but use them properly. Personalize books or handouts by writing in specific comments for that particular patient or encourage the patient to do this himself. Make sure you know what the chart, slide, overhead, or book says before you use it. Make sure that projection equipment is working and that you know how to use it.

When explaining things to patients remember that the medical terminology we take for granted is not in widespread use. Avoid 'medspeak'. Say 'high blood-glucose level' rather than 'hyperglycaemia' or 'passing lots of water' rather than 'polyuria', 'fatty tissue under the skin' rather than 'subcutaneous adipose layer'.

Three-stage teaching

The person with newly-diagnosed diabetes is too frightened and over-whelmed to take in large amounts of information. They need a survival pack which allows them to cope with their condition for a few days or weeks (Table 4.1). The second stage of teaching gradually extends the knowledge until all the appropriate areas have been covered. The third stage revises and updates the knowledge.

Table 4.1 The survival pack: vital points to be discussed following diagnosis

The diagosis
Diabetes:
is long term but controllable
has symptoms that will be relieved rapidly
is not catching
is not immediately fatal!

Diet
Know what and how much to eat—in simple terms

Treatment
Either tablets or insulin if needed
If insulin, know the basic technology

Hazard warnings
Free prescriptions for those on tablets or insulin

Monitoring
Finger-prick blood glucose monitoring
(Start with urine testing in really nervous patients)

Carry
Diabetes card and glucose everywhere

Drivers
If a driver, tell DVLA and motor insurance company immediately

Implications
Immediate implications for work, family, or leisure activities

Contact
Provide details of whom to contact for help

Concerns
Any questions or concerns

Appointment
The next meeting

Marion was 54 and frightened. I spent 30 minutes explaining that she had diabetes and exactly what that meant. A diabetic diet and some tablets would make her feel much better. She seemed much more cheerful when she left the consulting room. 'Thank you for explaining, doctor,' she said, en route for the dietitian. Five minutes later the dietitian knocked at the door. 'This lady says she's not diabetic!'

Mike was 10 when he was diagnosed diabetic. He was terrified. It was not until some years later that he confessed that because the word sounded like die, he thought he would do just that.

The details of each of these stages are covered in subsequent chapters.

Extending the patient's knowledge in several sessions

Most important in each session, answer the patient's questions; until you have done this they may not listen to the information which you wish to pass on.

Topics for further discussion include:

1. The causes of diabetes. How the pancreas works. Basic biochemistry of glucose, insulin, and fat. Inheritance of diabetes.

2. Check knowledge of dietary principles. Give more detailed dietary information.

3. Check tablet knowledge or insulin injection technique. How the treatment works. How to adjust it at home. More sophisticated regimens and equipment.

4. Check blood glucose measuring technique. Controlling the blood glucose and use of more sophisticated monitoring techniques.

5. Can they show you their diabetic card and glucose?

6. Have they told the relevant bodies or contacted self-help groups such as Diabetes UK?

7. Work, family, and leisure more detail (see Chapters 12–16).

8. How the diabetes team works. How to make the best use of this resource.

9. Body maintenance to maintain health and prevent tissue damage. The implications of diabetes and its complications.

10. The next meeting.

Revision

Studies suggest that skills and knowledge decline rapidly after training. They need updating regularly—perhaps every six months. If we do not check that patients have retained the information we think we have taught them, and, more to the point, that they are using it correctly, major misunderstandings and errors can occur.

Sue, an intelligent young woman with insulin-treated diabetes, was supposed to be injecting fast-acting Actrapid three times a day and long-acting Ultratard at night. That was what was written in her notes on each visit. Her blood glucose diary showed gross glucose fluctuations. On probing the reasons for this erratic control the doctor discovered that she was taking both Actrapid and Ultratard three times a day. It was clear that she had never understood the principles behind her original insulin regimen.

Another problem is that friends, relatives, the next-door neighbour, the man in the post office, are often more likely to be believed than the professionals.

Mavis was losing weight. She often showed urinary ketones. 'My friend's grandfather was diabetic. She said I should never touch starch. Fatal, you see, for a diabetic. Makes sugar. So I'm always very strict. No bread, no biscuits, no potato ever.'

Sometimes a little knowledge can be a very dangerous thing.

John was admitted to hospital with severe hypoglycaemia. He had had a hypoglycaemic episode but collapsed while trying to eat glucose. His neighbour, an ardent first aider, heard the crash, rushed in, and diagnosed a 'diabetic coma'. Surrounded by admiring relatives he injected a large amount of insulin into John's leg.

Even the most experienced patient (or diabetes care professional) should have their insulin administration and blood glucose monitoring techniques checked regularly. And even in the best-run clinic, information gaps occur. It is common to discover people who have not informed the DVLA of their insulin-treated diabetes—many years after diagnosis. And why is the diabetes card and glucose always in the other coat?

Co-ordinating diabetes education

The best person to co-ordinate diabetes education is the diabetes specialist nurse. Every person with diabetes should have access to a nurse with this special training. A chart in the patient's record, preferably the one they themselves hold, can be used to check off items and who has taught them. It is a humbling experience for many doctors to discover that patients are often more likely to remember what the nurse has taught them than their doctor's advice.

The diabetes team should get together and agree a consistent approach to all aspects of diabetes education. It is vital that the patient is not confused. This consistency should extend to all involved in patient care—general practitioners, other hospital staff, school teachers. If there is a divergence of opinion a national consensus may have been reached—ask Primary Care Diabetes UK.

Primary Care Diabetes UK provides a wide range of information for professionals and for people with diabetes. It is a multidisciplinary group of practitioners working in primary care who share a common interest in diabetes. Patients now have a clear idea of standards of care from the national and European patients' charters (Chapter 22).

Summary

- A person with diabetes must understand what diabetes is and how it may affect him.
- In diabetes it is primarily the person who has it who determines the outcome.
- The professionals must provide him or her with the knowledge and the tools to monitor his or her condition and to adjust treatment.

- ◆ Knowledge should be provided as and when the patient wants it, tailoring the professionals' agenda to the patient's individual needs.
- ◆ Knowledge should be consistent and teaching should be professional.
- ◆ Provide frequent revision sessions and support whenever it is required.
- ◆ Use the existing literature and professional support.

Chapter 5

Eating and drinking

A diet is what you eat. It is important to convey this to patients who may equate all diets with weight loss. While many people with diabetes do need to lose weight, a healthy diet should not be seen solely as a short-term means of losing a few pounds. It is a lifelong eating plan. Most people will start enthusiastically, spurred on by their anxieties about their new diabetes. However, the initial enthusiasm tends to lapse and many patients regain weight. It is important that people continue to enjoy their food and that the treatment of their diabetes is adjusted to their usual eating pattern and not *vice versa*.

The two parts of the diet are what you eat and how much.

What to eat

Current advice is that, of the total calories eaten, 55 per cent should be carbohydrate, less than 30–35 per cent should be fat, and 10–15 per cent should be protein (Fig. 5.1). Most people have no idea what this actually looks like on a plate. Fat supplies about twice the calories (9 kcal/g) as the same weight of protein (4 kcal/g) or carbohydrate (3.8 kcal/g). Food also contains water, fibre, and inedible waste such as orange peel. If a man working as a builder eats about 3000 kcal a day he may have 1000 kcal for his evening meal. Table 5.1 shows how this is translated into real food.

The builder's helpings of beans and vegetables are large, those of chicken, custard, and pie are small. This size of meal is only appropriate for an energetic young man. It would constitute the food for an entire day for an overweight person on a 1000 calorie diet. Forty per cent of the calories are in the sweet pudding in which a lot of fat is concealed in the pastry which also greatly increases the carbohydrate intake. For someone with diabetes it would have been better to have fruit alone. There is plenty of fibre in this meal—in the baked beans, potatoes, cabbage, and apple.

It took me some time to calculate this example and it is clearly unrealistic to expect our builder to sit down with the calculator and weighing scales before he tucks into his well-earned dinner. The simplest option is to encourage people with diabetes to learn about the different types of food. They should eat as much as they want of low-calorie foods such as green vegetables, large helpings of starchy, high-fibre carbohydrate foods, tiny helpings of fat, and moderate helpings of protein. Sugar and salt should be treated as rare treats or avoided. 'Made-up foods' not produced at home to a diabetes recipe should be viewed with suspicion as they often contain a lot of hidden sugar and fat (e.g. pies, sausages, cakes). The total amount eaten can be adjusted by the number of meals and snacks and the size of helpings—our builder could serve his food with a tablespoon and eat three big meals and three snacks a day, an overweight

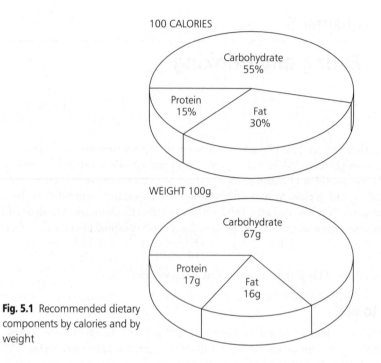

100 CALORIES

Carbohydrate
55%

Protein
15%

Fat
30%

WEIGHT 100g

Carbohydrate
67g

Protein
17g

Fat
16g

Fig. 5.1 Recommended dietary components by calories and by weight

typist could serve her food with a teaspoon and eat three small meals a day, with a bedtime snack if on insulin.

Table 5.1 The builder's meal (calculated from figures in the *Manual of nutrition*, 1989)

Food	Weight (g)	kcal	Protein (g)	Fat (g)	Carbohydrate (g)
Tomato soup	200	110	1.6	6.6	11.8
Roast chicken (meat)	100	148	24.8	5.4	0
Cabbage	200	30	3.4	0	4.6
Baked beans	200	162	9.6	1.2	30.2
Boiled potato	200	152	3.6	0.2	36.0
Apple pie[*]	100	369	4.3	15.5	56.7
Custard[*]	30	35	1.1	1.3	144.3
Total	1030	1006	48.4	30.2	144.3
kcal		1006	193	272	541
Percent of total kcal		100%	19%	27%	54%

[*] Made with sugar; full-fat milk in the custard. He drank mineral water with the meal.

Carbohydrate—starchy, sugary foods

The days of low-carbohydrate diets are long gone—or should be. There are still some patients who adhere to a crumpled and faded low-carbohydrate diet sheet.

Refined carbohydrate—sugar and glucose

Most people know that people with diabetes should reduce their sugar intake. Glucose and sucrose (the latter being digested into glucose) provide rapidly-absorbed carbohydrate. When eaten alone, this produces an abrupt rise in blood glucose concentration, detectable within minutes and continuing over the next two hours. Normally this is a stimulus for pancreatic insulin release which parallels the blood glucose rise. This cannot happen with an insulin depot in the subcutaneous tissue which does not enter the circulation fast enough.

However, when sucrose is eaten as part of a meal, the blood glucose rise following that meal is no greater than a meal of the same caloric value without sucrose. Better compliance may be achieved if patients are allowed a sweet with the lunch or after-dinner coffee, or if they are allowed to eat sucrose-containing puddings occasionally.

In insulin-treated patients, exercising vigorously, liver glucose release may not keep up with glucose uptake by muscles. The blood glucose can fall precipitously if the patient does not top up with sugar or glucose (see p. 118). Thus insulin-treated patients must understand that they can use sugar-containing foods when exercising. Regular exercise may eventually be fuelled mainly by unrefined carbohydrates.

> Damien had been diagnosed diabetic for only a few months when he attended an Outward Bound course. He was the only diabetic on the course. He had not told his physician that he was going and knew little about diabetes and nothing about diabetes and exercise. But he was confident about his diet. NO SUGAR. NO. NONE AT ALL. So when he went on expedition he filled his rucksack with apples. But the sucrose they contained was not enough. He collapsed with hypoglycaemia and his group, much alarmed, had to revive him with sweet tea. After this he accepted that it was all right to have sugary foods to provide fuel for prolonged and unaccustomed exercise.

The other occasion when sugar or glucose is essential is in the treatment of hypoglycaemia. Obvious? Not necessarily. If you tell the patient no sugar, he may obey you to the letter, fighting off all attempts to treat hypoglycaemia with sugar lumps.

Unrefined carbohydrate—starchy foods

Over half the dietary calories should come from starchy carbohydrates. This is a lot of carbohydrate. Ideally it should be mixed with fibre. Insoluble fibre such as wheat bran and the fibres found in vegetables like celery and cabbage helps to bulk out the food and make it filling, for example wholemeal bread, wholemeal pasta, brown rice, and potatoes in their jackets. Soluble fibre such as that found in beans and pulses has a more pronounced beneficial effect on digestion and absorption of carbohydrate. If possible everyone with diabetes should eat some beans, lentils, chick peas, or other pulse every day.

More people are used to a high-fibre diet nowadays, but if someone is making a radical change in their diet, introduce the new foods slowly to reduce abdominal griping and flatulence. It is better to take six months and achieve eventual dietary compliance, than to take six days and achieve permanent dietary rejection.

Carbohydrate portions

For years, people with insulin-treated diabetes (and sometimes those on oral hypoglycaemic drugs) were encouraged to weigh or measure carbohydrate portions. These are usually expressed in 10 g equivalents of carbohydrate. But, while this may give a general guide to carbohydrate quantities, there are several fallacies underlying this method. For example, the same food prepared in different ways will release its carbohydrate at different rates. An apple contains about 10 g carbohydrate. Eaten raw this carbohydrate will be available less readily than if the same apple was cooked, and will provide less readily available carbohydrate than if the apple was converted into apple juice. The same food eaten with various other foods will be absorbed at different rates (for example, fats slow absorption). What the patient is doing—resting, exercising—and the state of their heart and vasculature, will influence the blood supply to the gut and hence the rise in blood glucose after food.

The glycaemic index compares the area under the blood glucose curve after eating a particular food with that after eating an equivalent amount of carbohydrate as glucose. Using this technique an apple has a glycaemic index (expressed as a percentage) of 39, baked beans 40, brown rice 66, wholemeal bread 72, honey 87, and Lucozade 98; glucose is 100 per cent.

For practical purposes, it is helpful if patients on insulin treatment know roughly how much carbohydrate different foods contain as it will help them to work out their insulin dose, but there is no reason nowadays to make them weigh their food and calculate exact grams of carbohydrate. The carbohydrate foods should be spread out in three meals a day, convenient for the patient. If they are taking insulin, a coffee-time and teatime snack is desirable, and a bedtime snack can be essential. Overweight patients not on insulin should avoid snacks.

Fruit and vegetables

We should eat five portions of fruit or vegetables a day. Fruit tastes sweet because it contains sucrose and fructose. The sweeter it tastes the more refined carbohydrate it contains. So grapes contain a lot of sucrose. Fruit is an important source of vitamin C. But if fruit is eaten in large amounts it will cause an elevation in blood glucose and in weight.

Vegetables can be divided into two groups. Those which can be eaten in large amounts with little influence on weight or carbohydrate, and those which have to be considered as an energy source. Leafy vegetables such as lettuce and cabbage, big watery containers of small seeds like tomato, cucumber, and courgette, and swollen stalks such as celery, leeks, and onions can be eaten with impunity. Very fibrous root vegetables like carrots and turnip contain only small amounts of carbohydrate entangled in the fibre. Starchy root vegetables such as potatoes, and big seeds, for example beans, peas, lentils, other pulses, and nuts contain a lot of carbohydrate to fuel the growing plant after germination. They need to be considered in carbohydrate totals.

Fats—greasy, oily foods

Less than 35 per cent of dietary calories should come from fat. This is a very small amount of visible fat because so much is concealed in other foods, especially manufactured. Fat makes food taste good and few people realize how calorific it is. The pat of butter contains the same number of calories as the slice of bread on which it is spread.

Naked fat is relatively easy to avoid. Tell the patient to spread the butter thinly, or better still go without or change to less fatty meats such as skinned chicken or turkey. Avoid hard cheese, cream cheeses, and lard or dripping. Avoid cream and use semi-skimmed milk or skimmed milk. Avoid fried foods. Do not use oil-based salad dressings.

Hidden fat can most readily be avoided by self-catering. Do not add fat to cooking unless essential—there are plenty of low-fat cookery books to choose from. But many of us do not have the time or the desire to cook complex recipes. So advise patients to read the information on the packet. Increasingly foods are being marketed in fat-reduced form but beware, such products may still be high in fat. For example, half the calories in lower-fat crisps still come from fat. Meat products (sausages, salami, pork pies, beefburgers) are very high in fat.

Saturated, monounsaturated, and polyunsaturated fats

So much attention is paid to the type of fat that the overriding principle of total fat reduction tends to be forgotten. People feel very virtuous eschewing butter and choosing polyunsaturated margarine. But margarine, must, by definition, contain 80 per cent fat so it should still be used sparingly. Much of the fat which is eaten should be in the form of monounsaturates (e.g. olive oil, avocado pear) and polyunsaturates (such as sunflower oil). Dairy and meat fats are mostly saturated and should be reduced in quantity.

Protein

If 50–60 per cent of the dietary calories are carbohydrate and 30 per cent are fat, that only leaves 10–20 per cent as protein. That is the equivalent of about 150 g of chicken meat (5 oz) on a 1500 calorie diet. Because many proteins are closely associated with fat, white meat, fish, and vegetable protein (e.g. soya), with some low-fat cheese and one or two eggs a week should be the main protein source. Red meat should be lean and grilled or casseroled rather than roasted or fried.

Salt

Sodium chloride has long been linked with hypertension and may worsen fluid retention in oedematous patients. Patients should be advised not to add salt at table and to use it sparingly in cooking (unless exercising in hot weather or participating in endurance sports).

Drinks

Tea and coffee may be the vehicles for full fat milk or cream and sugar. As some people drink six to eight cups of tea a day, this can include a pint of milk and large quantities of sugar. Semi-skimmed milk and artificial sweeteners such as aspartame can help the patient towards skimmed milk and no sweetener (or even black tea or coffee).

Aerated 'diet' drinks containing artificial sweeteners can be drunk in moderation. Care is needed in reading the labels of some products marked 'sugar-free' which may contain other refined carbohydrates, for example glucose.

Savoury drinks used to be encouraged but most of these are very salty.

Alcohol

Moderation in all things. The recommended amount is 14 units a week for a woman and 21 units a week for a man. A unit is half a pint of beer, lager, or cider, a single pub measure of spirits, or a glass of wine. So 21 units is 1.5 pints each night. Alcohol is highly calorific ranging from 285 calories per unit for sweet cider to 50 calories per unit for spirits.

Much confusion is generated by the carbohydrate content of alcoholic drinks. Very sweet drinks should be avoided, but otherwise there is no particular benefit in using low-carbohydrate products (e.g. beers) as the carbohydrate has been turned to alcohol by further brewing. Although the total calorie content should be considered if the patient needs to lose weight, it is better to ignore the carbohydrate contribution of alcoholic drinks.

Alcohol impedes glucose release from liver glycogen stores and may precipitate or worsen hypoglycaemia. I advise people with diabetes never to drink on an empty stomach. A packet of crisps or preferably another lower-fat snack, if available, should be consumed if alcohol is drunk outside mealtimes.

'Diabetic' products

Diabetes UK has now banned advertising of these products from its magazine. They are sweets, biscuits, and cakes in which glucose and sucrose have been replaced by fructose or sorbitol. There is no evidence that fructose is any better for diabetics than sucrose and it may be metabolically worse. Sorbitol, which is the other commonly used sweetener, causes abdominal griping and diarrhoea when consumed in large amounts. Many of these products are highly calorific. Patients should be discouraged from buying them.

How much to eat

As much as is necessary to reach and maintain normal weight and fuel physical activity.

Most people have difficulty applying the principles of energy balance to them-selves—the author included. The concept that, to maintain weight, energy input should balance the energy used and that to lose weight, energy consumed should be less than energy expended, is rarely difficult to transmit. The problem is that few people realize how little energy they use and what it represents in terms of food on the plate. And when they do learn this, they yet may be unable to resist eating more. Unfortunately appetite is no guide as food is used for so many other purposes than simple survival. Western society encourages generous portions and failure visibly to enjoy food by eating it all is considered an insult to its provider. Children are often admonished or even punished for failing to eat up everything on their plates. 'You must eat up, think of all the starving people abroad,' said one mother. 'Well, it would be no good to them because it would all go rotten in the post,' reasoned the child as he pushed his plate away. So we eat more than we actually want to comply with parental or society pressure. In other circumstances we use food as a comforter or just as something to do. Many people have fallen into the habit of nibbling while watching television and sales of savoury snacks are booming.

Convey quantities of different types of food in a way which is readily understood and allows people to manage their own diet without application to a calculator. There is rarely any need to count calories. They are a general guide only, as myriad factors influence energy availability from a particular food prepared in a particular way for a particular individual. Do you know what 100 calories of brown bread looks like? It is a large slice. 100 calories of butter is a small pat.

Obesity

Many patients with Type 2 diabetes are obese. There is no simple answer to the management of obesity. Most of the patients I see know that they weigh too much, and many have tried to lose weight. The aim is a body mass index between 18 and 25 kg/m^2.

What are they eating already? A dietary diary (underline the importance of honesty) for a week can be a helpful guide if the patient wishes to comply. Otherwise take a dietary history.

Modify the type of foods eaten Reducing fat and alcohol can help considerably as they are both highly calorific.

Reduce the quantities eaten Although many obese people claim not to eat excessive amounts, observing some of them in self-service restaurants shows their portion sizes are larger than other peoples. Using a smaller spoon to serve with and putting the food onto a smaller plate so that it looks more can help. Other overweight people genuinely do eat moderate amounts—they need to eat even less. (Patients are greatly insulted by the suggestion that they are greedy. Once antagonized a patient is less ready to accept future advice.) Another suggestion that sometimes helps is to remove a teaspoonful of food from each portion and put it back, or throw it away. (It is more acceptable, and more economical, to start with less food as many of those who lived through the war get very upset at the idea of wasting food, even when it is better for an overweight person to throw it away than to eat it!)

When is the food eaten? Habit eating, for example while watching television, while driving (dangerous), while working at a desk, while serving behind the counter, while chatting, are all times when the food may be put in the mouth, chewed, and swallowed with little appreciation of its flavour. Substitute calorie-free chewing gum or a minimum calorie drink.

Why do people eat? Fat people need to eat very little to survive. Appetite can overcome satiety—we can be completely full of meat and vegetables but still fancy a piece of chocolate gateau. Food is a great comforter. It is an excuse for a social or family gathering. It is an expression of welcome, a thank you present, a sign that you care. It is sometimes used as a weapon—'Eat up your greens.' 'Shan't.' 'Eat them up, there's a good girl.' 'No, I won't.' 'Go on, try a little bit.' 'No, no, NO.' Eating may simply be something to do with your hands. Find out why your patient is eating the foods he or she eats and suggest substitution of another activity or lower calorie foods as appropriate.

Where is the food eaten and with whom? Eating alone allows unwitnessed greed and dietary sinning. Eating with a bad influence can encourage dietary sinning. The 'naughty but nice' advertising campaign for cream focused on this feeling of wickedness—no one actually likes being good all the time. Eating pre-packed food or food produced in a staff canteen can destroy dietary effort. If all the works canteen stocks is pork pies and chips, there is little hope for the diet unless the patient takes a packed lunch.

> Hamish works in an airport. Everyday he has to pass through the security section to get to work. Everything he carries has to go through the X-ray machine. 'I have to eat the food they give us at work because I can't eat X-rayed sandwiches,' he said when I asked why his weight had gone up again. Reassurance that the wholesomeness of his diabetic diet would be unimpaired by X-rays was not well received.

Home-cooked meals may prove difficult if the cook is not the person with diabetes and does not understand dietary requirements. Wives usually change their diet to suit their husband's diabetic diet. A husband rarely changes his diet if his wife has diabetes.

Read the packet Most foods now have detailed content and calorie lists. But few packs weigh exactly 100 g. And what is a gram anyway? Many British cooks still think in pounds and ounces. 100 g is 3.5 oz. One ounce is about 30 g.

Introducing a diet

People want recognition of the difficulties of finding the will-power to lose weight and of their needs to have the occasional forbidden food. With this approach the overall goal is discussed—but a reasonable interim goal is set in agreement with the patient. Failure to meet the goal is ignored; success, however slight, must be praised enthusiastically. Success breeds success.

Sometimes group support helps, as in Weight Watchers, where there is also a financial incentive. Enlisting a family member to watch the diet and give encouragement may help for some people.

The patient needs to be able to monitor his or her own progress. Advise weekly weigh-ins, preferably by someone else, at the same time of day and in the same clothes, with the result written on a graph.

Some advisers favour the authoritarian approach. 'You are two stone overweight. Here is your diet sheet. You must stick to it or I will be very cross with you. Come and see me in three months.' Three months later if the patient has gained weight—'You are a very bad girl, go away and try harder'; or lost weight—'well done, good girl. Keep up the good work.' The patient who gains weight is accused of not trying hard enough. Many patients are insulted by being treated as children and they resent the implication that they are not trying. They vote with their feet and do not reattend.

There is no easy formula to help people lose weight—the one constant factor of most studies is that continued interest and support is helpful.

It is easy to sit in a consulting room pontificating about the patient's diet. However, it may be very hard for the patient to put our glibly delivered advice into practice. The patient should be told the best option—a weight-normalizing, high-carbohydrate, high-fibre, low-sugar, low-fat diet—and then be encouraged to have a realistic discussion of the sort of diet they feel able to achieve. Relatives and carers should be involved. In some instances, especially with elderly people, the goal may simply be to eat something every day.

> Bert, 84, and treated with oral hypoglycaemic agents, was admitted with pneumonia. A history was unobtainable because he was also hypoglycaemic. As he recovered the nurses had great difficulty persuading him to eat his meals. It transpired that he ate a breakfast of bread and jam, but no lunch or evening meal at home. He rejected meals on wheels. He was eventually admitted to a long-stay ward.
>
> Frederick, 75, was arthritic and had cerebrovascular disease. He had insulin-treated diabetes. He received meals on wheels daily, carefully prepared to be suitable for a diabetic diet. He reported frequent hypoglycaemia at clinic and his insulin was reduced. Some weeks later, the meals on wheels co-ordinator contacted the clinic to ask if Fred could have ordinary meals—he was leaving his carefully prepared diabetic food untouched. He is now well and happy on a non-diabetic diet and the hypoglycaemia has stopped.

Different diets

Vegetarians often find a healthy diet easy. They may well be following it anyway. If they are vegans, protein can be obtained from vegetable sources (such as quorn, pulses, nuts). Vegans may become deficient in vitamin B_{12}, requiring replacement therapy. Lacto-vegetarians may need to use lower-fat dairy products.

It is vital to be sensitive to religious dietary requirements. Limitations on meats are rarely a problem in working out the diabetic diet, but the traditional ways of cooking may use a lot of fat (ghee for example). Brown rice or wholemeal flour can be substituted for lower-fibre products (but remember that to eat white rice may reflect higher status). Although the rural diets of peoples in South Asia and Africa are high-fibre and low-sugar, this does not necessarily apply to the urban diet, particularly that adopted by people who have emigrated to Britain. Unless the person who actually cooks the patient's food sees the dietitian or diabetes team it is unlikely that dietary advice given in the surgery will succeed (see p. 176).

Fast days or periods of denial occur in many religions, both Eastern and Western. Ramadan places particular demands on insulin-treated patients. Most religious leaders will exempt a diabetic from this religious observance, but the patient may feel participation to be essential for spiritual well-being. Sometimes meals are eaten during the hours of darkness and attention should be given to long-lasting carbohydrate with plenty of fibre in the last meal before dawn. Insulin doses must be adjusted to cope with the long period without food.

Never underestimate the strength of a person's belief in the rightness of their traditional diet. Many hours of explanation may be needed to convince the patient that the new diabetic diet is better for them.

Eating out and abroad

> Nadia and her husband enjoyed eating out. Then Nadia developed diabetes. She followed her diet meticulously. She was afraid that she would eat the wrong foods in restaurants. So she and her husband stayed in. But her husband became increasingly annoyed about this. A rift developed in their marriage. Nadia spent a week with a group of people with diabetes enjoying outdoor activities. Meals were varied and she also learned how other participants coped with their diets. Back home, she and her husband began to eat out again and harmony was restored.

People with diabetes need not avoid other people's cooking. The occasional non-diet meal is not a disaster. However, if they eat out often, some common sense is necessary. A reasonable meal could be a starter of melon or consomme, a main course of grilled fish or grilled steak, or chicken (cut the skin off), with baked or boiled potatoes and vegetables or salad, followed by fruit. Avoid sauces and roast dishes, limit alcohol, and limit the sweet trolley.

Emergency foods

Everyone taking insulin injections or other glucose-lowering medication, should keep a store of emergency food to substitute for a missed meal. It should be durable, conveniently packaged, and easy to carry around. The wide range of muesli and high-fibre bars are ideal as they contain some starchy carbohydrate and some sucrose mixed with plenty of fibre. They fit in a pocket, handbag, or workbox and can be left lying in a desk drawer or under the dashboard of the car for months. Small boxes of fruit juice, nuts, and raisins, and packs of savoury snacks are all useful.

Eating disorders in diabetes

Perhaps because of the constant emphasis on food and diet in diabetes, eating disorders are more common than is realized. Eating disorders associated with diabetes range from restriction of carbohydrate or omitting meals to reduce the blood glucose to a more sinister severe carbohydrate restriction to reduce the insulin dose and reduce weight. Some anorexic patients deliberately induce insulin deficiency and hyperglycaemia to lose weight. They tend to be admitted in biochemical chaos and ketoacidosis. (Laxative abuse and insulin deficiency cause dangerous hypokalaemia.) Anorexia nervosa may alternate with bulimia. Bulimia produces gross fluctuations in glucose balance as the overeating may need large insulin doses, but the self-induced vomiting then precipitates hypoglycaemia. Such patients should be referred to a specialist diabetes service and be seen in conjunction with psychiatric and psychological support. Abnormal eating patterns may persist for many years before being detected and some people with diabetes never again have a normal attitude to food.

Dietary advice

Every patient should see a dietitian on diagnosis of diabetes and annually thereafter. There is a tendency for many patients to assume that there is no need to worry about the diet if they are taking their diabetes tablets or insulin. The diabetic diet is an integral part of treatment and medical staff must ensure that patients realize this. All those caring for people with diabetes should be aware of dietary requirements and be able to answer questions about food.

Summary

- ◆ A diet is what you eat. Teach patients about the types of food and the amounts of food to eat.
- ◆ A healthy diet should be high-carbohydrate, high-fibre, low-sugar, low-fat, and low-salt, with alcohol in moderation.
- ◆ In the obese Type 2 patient weight reduction is the most important part of treatment.
- ◆ All patients should achieve normal weight for their height.
- ◆ Try to strike a balance between practicality and theory. Use common sense and do not forget that patients are people.
- ◆ Adapt the treatment to the patient, not the patient to the treatment.

Suggested reading

Ministry of Agriculture, Fisheries, and Food (1989). *Manual of nutrition*. Her Majesty's Stationery Office, London.

Nutrition Subcommittee of the British Diabetic Association's Professional Advisory Committee (1991). Dietary recommendations for people with diabetes: an update for the 1990s. *Journal of Human Nutrition and Dietetics*, **4**, 393–412.

Chapter 6

Urine monitoring

Glucose, protein (albumin), and ketones can all be monitored simply in urine. Urine glucose testing was the mainstay of diabetes self care, but is now used less often.

The person testing the urine must

- understand why they are doing the test
- be capable of following instructions
- not be colour blind
- not suffer visual impairment
- not have impeding upper-limb disabilities.

Urine glucose monitoring

Who should test?

Health care professionals as a simple, non-invasive screening measure. Because of the variation in renal threshold, absence of glycosuria does not exclude diabetes. Similarly, glycosuria does not prove diabetes, although it is suggestive and should be followed up. Postprandial testing is more likely to detect diabetes than fasting samples. Up to 15 per cent of pregnant women show glycosuria, but most of these do not have diabetes.

People with diabetes or their carers as a first step to learning about self-monitoring, or as their only means of self-monitoring. Ideally, urine glucose monitoring should be used only after urinalyses during an oral glucose tolerance test or blood glucose series have demonstrated the renal threshold. The threshold is usually about 10 mmol/l. Urine glucose monitoring is too imprecise for most insulin-treated patients and should not be used as the sole means of testing in any patients capable and willing to measure finger-prick blood glucose. Some physicians advocate urine testing for well-controlled Type 2 patients and blood testing for Type 1 patients. While there may be less rapid fluctuations in blood glucose concentration in Type 2 diabetes, it is helpful for patients to have an accurate knowledge of their blood glucose status. Some patients like to use both blood and urine testing.

Table 6.1 Testing urine for glucose

Mid-stream

Take an in-date bottle of urine testing strips

Remove one strip and close the bottle firmly

Hold the strip briefly in the urine stream

Start timing immediately

Tap off the excess urine

Compare the colour with the chart on that bottle the instant the time is up

Saved sample

Save the sample in a sterile urine bottle—wide-topped is easiest. (Do not use a half-rinsed pickle jar)

Test as soon as possible after passing

Dip the strip in the urine

Start timing immediately

Tap off the excess

Compare the colour with the chart on the bottle the instant the time is up

When to test for glycosuria

To monitor the overnight blood glucose balance, test the first urine passed on rising in the morning. For a fasting, pre-breakfast test, empty the bladder on rising, then test a specimen voided 30 to 60 minutes later, but before eating. Patients need to be reminded that the concentration of glucose in the urine depends upon the height of the blood glucose above the renal threshold during the period since last voiding (often many hours) and the volumes of fluid passed. Many patients think that the urine glucose now, reflects the blood glucose now. The results should be written down, with an indication of the period covered.

Urine versus blood glucose testing

The pros No needles, no finger-pricks, no risk of infection to the tested and minimal risk of infection to testers. Simple equipment—just a bottle of strips—which is easy to use.

The cons The method is dependent upon renal threshold which varies from person to person and over time in one individual.

A lavatory or other appropriate place is essential. It is retrospective, and it is difficult to make immediate adjustments to insulin dose. If there is no glucose in the urine the patient does not know whether his blood glucose is normal, or whether he is hypoglycaemic—hence the old advice to keep a trace of glucose in the urine (which meant, in practice, keeping the blood glucose over 10 mmol/l, hardly normoglycaemia).

Aspirin and vitamin C interfere with urine glucose testing, giving false negative results.

Ketones

Ketones are a product of fat breakdown; their presence in urine is a sign of insulin deficiency. However, anything which causes major fat breakdown, such as a strict weight-reducing diet, will cause ketonuria. Some patients have been much frightened by the teaching that ketonuria always indicates impending coma. Ketone testing strips are available in bottles and individually foil wrapped. The latter are better for patient use as they keep better and most patients need them infrequently. (Finger-prick ketone-testing strips may soon be available.)

When to test for ketones

New patients Always test the urine of a newly diagnosed diabetic for ketones: if present in large amounts they indicate the need for insulin treatment.

Ill insulin-treated patients May well have relative insulin deficiency and should be encouraged to test for ketones. This is especially important if they are vomiting or are short of breath. Such patients who present to their doctor must have a urine ketone test.

Very high blood glucose Patients should test for ketones if their blood glucose concentration is over 25 mmol/l (or outside the range of their meter), even if otherwise well.

Albumin

Everyone loses some albumin in their urine—in fit adults the loss ranges between 2.5 and 11 mg per 24 hours. Within a 24-hour period the excretion rate varies depending on, for example, posture and exertion. Protein excretion above 25 mg per 24 hours is not only a marker for the development of diabetic nephropathy but also, in Type 2 diabetes, for early mortality (mostly from cardiovascular causes). Efforts are therefore being made to detect small increases in proteinuria at an early stage. This is called microalbuminuria. Albustix will detect 300 mg/l albumin in urine; this is not sensitive enough for sufficiently early detection. More sensitive strips are now available to test for microalbuminuria.

During a normal night in which the patient is fully rested less than 30 μg albumin should be passed per minute. A timed overnight urine sample in which the urinary albumin concentration has been corrected for urinary creatinine concentration is probably the most accurate and reproducible estimation. But this presents some difficulties in ordinary practice. One answer is to ask patients to bring in early morning specimens of urine on which the albumin/creatinine ratio should be below 3.5 in women and below 2.5 in men. This does mean that the sample has to be sent to the laboratory. Another method is to ask the patient to bring in a large bottle containing all the urine passed overnight and dip-stick test it for microalbumin. The albumin concentration should be below 20 mg/l.

Cetrimide (as in Savlon) and chlorhexidine (e.g. Hibitane) can give a false positive result. False positives may also be found in concentrated urine.

When to test for albumin

All newly-diagnosed patients Should have an Albustix urine test. If this is negative, microalbumin should be measured.

All patients Should have their urine albumin checked annually using a microalbumin technique. If they already have proteinuria detectable using Albustix there is no need for the more sensitive test.

Patients with microalbuminuria If microalbuminuria is confirmed on two further tests during the next month prescribe ACE inhibitor treatment. Repeat tests after intervention to monitor their progress.

Summary

◆ Urine glucose testing of postprandial samples can be used to detect diabetes (beware false negatives and false positives).

◆ Urine glucose testing can be used to monitor glycaemic balance but is less reliable than blood glucose testing.

◆ Urine ketone testing should be used to detect the need for insulin therapy in newly-diagnosed patients. It may indicate the need for increased insulin dosage in those who are ill or markedly hyperglycaemic.

◆ Urine albumin testing should detect small amounts of albumin and thus micro-albumin measurement is preferable to Albustix. Urine microalbumin testing detects patients at risk of worsening nephropathy at a stage when intervention may slow the rate of progression. It also warns of increased risk of cardiovascular mortality in Type 2 patients.

Further reading

NICE (2002). Management of Type 2 diabetes. Renal disease-prevention and early management. Inherited Clinical Guideline F. *www.nice.org.uk*

Chapter 7

Blood glucose testing

Blood glucose testing includes capillary blood glucose monitoring from finger-prick samples, laboratory estimation of venous plasma (or whole blood) glucose, or retrospective measures using glycosylated proteins—fructosamine and haemoglobin $A1_c$.

Laboratory estimation

This is the gold standard against which other methods are compared. When taking venous blood, note the time in the patient's records and ensure that the bottle is not over-filled or under-filled. Mix it gently. Label the bottle and the form for the correct patient. Same-day analysis is best, but if this is not possible, the sample can be kept in a 4° refrigerator. Enter the results in your record, tell the patient, and act as outlined below. Temper these guidelines with your knowledge of the individual patient. (See Tables 8.1 and 9.1)

Results of laboratory venous plasma glucose estimation

1 < 2.2 mmol/l. Inform the patient of the test results on the same day. Did you or the patient realize that they were hypoglycaemic at the time? If not the patient needs to know that they have hypoglycaemic unawareness. And you need to sharpen your clinical observation. It is always possible for you to detect the subtle signs of hypoglycaemia if you are thinking about it. Unless it was a one-off low, their treatment regimen should be changed. Telephone patients on medium- or long-acting oral hypoglycaemic drugs to make sure that they are not still hypoglycaemic.

2 2.2–3.9 mmol/l. Sailing a little close to the wind. In patients on sulphonylurea or insulin therapy consider reducing therapy or eating more (if not overweight).

3 4.0–6.9 mmol/l. Within normal limits; no action need be taken.

4 7.0–19.9 mmol/l. Not too good. Discuss eating less or increasing glucose-lowering treatment.

5 20 mmol/l or more. Much too high. Surprisingly, many patients tolerate blood glucose levels like this much of the time. Others will be very symptomatic or most unwell. Telephone the patient that day and check that they are all right. If the level is 30 mmol/l or more the patient should be seen by a doctor that day. They may need insulin and most need hospital admission. See Chapter 11.

Finger-prick capillary blood glucose testing

This is a more direct and precise way of monitoring blood glucose concentration than urine testing. Urine testing should not be used by professionals in hospitals or surgeries to monitor glycaemia in known diabetes. Among out-patients, all those capable of doing so and who wish to, should measure finger-prick blood glucose.

Who can use finger-prick glucose testing?

Professionals

The technique provides a rapid indication of the blood glucose without waiting for the laboratory. Providing the test is performed properly, the results are nearly as accurate as those obtained in the laboratory. However, the results are usually 13–15 per cent lower than a simultaneous venous plasma glucose measurement. If the user and the meter participate in a quality assurance scheme and have regular retraining, the results can be used for most diabetes management. Problems may arise when inexperienced personnel are asked to test blood glucose without any training. Every finger-prick glucose-testing problem investigated in one busy district general hospital was found to be due to user error.

People with diabetes or their relatives or carers

Finger-prick blood glucose testing has taken the guesswork out of life with diabetes. Patients no longer have to rely on urine tests and symptoms to manage their diabetes. Initially self-glucose monitoring was reserved for insulin-treated patients, but nowadays, every person with diabetes capable of performing the test should be monitoring their own blood glucose. Clearly, patients who have to make frequent adjustments to their insulin need to test more often than those on diet alone or on oral hypoglycaemics. However, enthusiasm for blood glucose testing should not allow carers to press its use in people for whom it is clearly inappropriate (see below). Those who do use it should be taught the technique properly, and given revision sessions.

The person testing the blood must:

- understand why they are doing the test
- be capable of following instructions
- not be colour blind unless using a meter
- not suffer visual impairment unless using a talking meter
- not have severe impeding upper-limb disabilities.

A woman in her 70s always recorded her blood glucose as 10 mmol/l. One day her doctor asked her to demonstrate. She pricked her finger, wiped the blood on to a piece of cotton wool, peered at it, said '10' and wrote the number down in her book.

Another elderly woman produced her blood glucose diary proudly—she tested several times every day. In the diary were scores of blood spots—neatly placed in the columns on the page. She had never understood what the bottle of little sticks was for.

How to do a finger-prick blood glucose test

Like all laboratory techniques performed outside the laboratory, finger-prick blood glucose measurement is a waste of time unless it is done properly. Important factors are:

- The finger
- Making the hole
- The blood drop
- The strips
- Timing
- Wiping/blotting
- Reading the result
- Recording the result
- Acting on the result
- Staff protection

The finger Should be warm, clean, and dry. Wash with water then dry. Sticky fingers give falsely high blood glucose levels. The sides of the finger are less sensitive than the tip. Some people also use their ear lobe.

Making the hole Lancets are for single use only and a fresh one is used each time. They can be used alone but spring-loaded finger-pricking devices are less painful e.g. Autolet or Soft-Touch. All these devices have platforms to press on to the finger. Use a new platform for each patient to avoid transmission of blood-borne infection. There are platforms of different thickness for deeper or shallower finger-prick. See Table 7.1(a).

The blood drop Should be allowed to form naturally. If necessary blood may be 'milked' up from the base of the finger. Squeezing the finger tip can dilute the blood with serum and may make the finger sore. The blood (not much, not too little) should be dropped onto the strip and never smeared.

The strips Must be in date and dry. Never handle the pad onto which the blood will be dropped—your sticky fingers might influence the result.

> I saw a woman with diabetes in a maternity hospital. I needed to check her blood glucose. The bottle of strips produced from the trolley was over a year out of date.

In one study of 46 general practices interested in diabetes care, five practices had the wrong strips for their blood glucose meter.

Timing Tests are usually done automatically by a meter. If not, a watch with a second hand is essential. If the test is not timed accurately the result is meaningless. Each strip has a different timing sequence which must be observed to the second.

Wiping or blotting In some strips (e.g. BM) the blood is wiped off the pad to allow the colour to be read after further timing. Cotton wool should be used as tissues scratch the surface and alter light reflectance. Other strips are blotted with a tissue. These techniques require practice as remaining blood will obviously affect the result.

Reading the result A properly-used meter is best. Each bottle of strips has a colour chart against which to match the colour changes of the strips in that bottle. (The dyes in each batch may change slightly so strips must not be matched against a bottle from a different batch.) The person reading the result must have normal colour vision. Colour blindness is a contraindication. People with diabetic retinopathy, especially those who have had laser treatment, may not have normal colour vision. People may not always understand what they are supposed to be reading.

Table 7.1(a) Finger prickers and compatible lancets

Compatible Lancets	Finger Pricking Devices*														
	Auto Lancet	Autolet	Autolet Lite	Autolet Mini	BD Lancer 5	BD Optimus	Glucoject	Glucolet	Hypolance	Microlet	Monojector	Penlet II	Prestige Smart System	Soft Touch	Softclix
BD Microfine +	●			●	●	●	●	●		●	●	●	●	●	
Finepoint	●				●	●		●	●	●		●	●	●	
GlucoTip			●	●	●	●	●	●	●	●			●	●	
Microlet	●	●	●	●	●	●		●	●	●	●	●	●	●	
Milward Steri-let	●	●	●	●	●	●	●	●	●	●	●	●	●	●	
Milward Steri-let Ultra Fine	●	●	●	●	●	●	●	●	●	●	●	●	●	●	
Monolet	●	●	●	●	●	●		●	●	●	●	●	●		
Monolet Extra		●	●										●		
One Touch Ultrasoft	●		●	●	●	●		●	●	●	●	●	●	●	
Softclix	●							●					●		●
Unilet GP	●	●				●							●		
Unilet Superlite	●		●				●						●		
Unilet GP Superlite	●	●	●	●	●	●	●	●	●	●	●	●	●	●	
Unilet Universal Comfort Touch	●	●	●	●	●	●	●	●	●	●	●	●	●	●	
Vitrex	●	●	●	●	●	●	●	●	●	●	●	●	●	●	

*N.B.: Finger pricking devices are not prescribable at NHS expense.

Reproduced from MIMS *Monthly Index of Medical Specialities* with permission. This table is updated every month; please see current issue for up-to-date information

Table 7.1(b) Blood glucose testing strips and meters

Meter	Sensitivity Range (mmol/l)	Company	Retail Price (exc. VAT)	Active	Advantage II	BM Accutest	BM Test 1–44	Glucometer Esprit Sensors	ExacTech	GlucoMen Test Sensors	Glucostix	Glucofide	Hypoguard Supreme	Hypoguard Supreme-reme Spectrum	MediSense G2	MediSense Optium	Medi-Test Glycaemic C	One Touch Ultra	Pocketscan	Prestige Smart System
Accu-Chek Active	0.6–33.3	Roche Diag.	£20.00	●																
Accu-Chek Advantage	0.6–33.3	Roche Diag.	£15.00		●															
Accutrend!	1.1–33.3	Roche Diag.	£34.00			●														
Accutrend GC*	1.1–33.3	Roche Diag.	£199.00			●														
Exac Tech	2.2–25	Medi Sense	£59.00						●											
GlucoMen Glyco	1.1–33.3	Menanni Diag.	£35.00							●										
Glucometer 2!	1–44	Bayer	–								●									
Glucometer 4!	0.6–33.3	Bayer	–								●									
Glucometer Esprit	0.6–33.3	Bayer	£24.99					●												
Glucometer GX!	1–44	Bayer	–									●								
Glucotrend 2!	0.6–33.3	Roche Diag.	£25.00	●																
Glucotrend Premium	0.56–33.3	Roche Diag.	£49.00	●																
Glycotronic C	1.1–33.3	BHR	£31.00														●			
Hypoguard Supreme Plus	2–22.0	Hypoguard (UK)	£35.00										●							
Hypoguard Supreme Extra	2–22.2	Hypoguard (UK)	£40.00										●							
MediSense Card	1.1–33.3	Medi Sense	£35.00												●					
MediSense Optium	1.1–33.3	Medi Sense	£45.00													●				
MediSense Pen	1.1–33.3	Medi Sense	£35.00												●					
Medisense Precision QID	1.1–33.3	Medi Sense	£35.00												●					
One Touch Ultra	1.1–33.3	Lifescan	£15.00															●		
PocketScan	1.1–33.3	Lifescan	£17.50																●	
Prestige Smart System	1.4–33.3	DiagnoSys Medical	£7.50																	●

● Meters are not available at NHS expense.
* Combined Glucose/Cholesterol Meter
! Meter no longer marketed

Reproduced from MIMS *Monthly Index of Medical Specialities* with permission. This table is updated every month; please see current issue for up-to-date information

One elderly couple tried to make words out of the numbers on the meter when I showed them a blood glucose result. Another woman read it upside-down—0.6 instead of 9.0. More seriously, a midwife refused to allow a hypoglycaemic woman to eat. 'Your glucose is 7, you don't need biscuits' she said. The biosensor actually read LO—the midwife had turned the device upside-down and read the result as 07. Fortunately, the patient just grabbed the biscuits and ate them. Warning messages may be misinterpreted—a nurse informed me that a patient had ketones in her blood. I asked how she had measured this. She told me it 'came up on the meter'. What the biosensor actually indicated was 'Check ketones'! A new meter does measure ketones.

Recording the result Many patients do not write their results down. While a one-off test may be of use at the time it was done, without a record neither the patient nor their carer can assess overall glucose balance and the need or otherwise for intervention. There may be other problems:

A young woman confidently presented her glucose diary to her doctor. A beautiful record, four tests a day, neatly written, all normal. The only problem was that she had filled in tomorrow's results as well!

There is a human tendency to under-read or to fail to record unpalatable results. But a substantial minority of patients make up their results to please their doctor. Fakes may be very tidy books, all written in the same pen at the same angle, often with the same numbers. (But some meticulous patients like to produce a clean copy of their rough results for their doctors.) A sophisticated faker may be detected only by repeated marked disparity between the glycosylated haemoglobin and home-recorded glucose levels.

Acting on the result It is no use noting an abnormal result and doing nothing about it. In one district general hospital audit, only one in four markedly abnormal blood glucose results recorded by nursing staff was acted upon. Patients frequently record very high or very low results for weeks without taking action.

Protecting staff Four or five finger-stick injuries due to glucose testing were reported each year to the occupational health unit in one hospital. Many more occur but are not reported. There is an obvious risk of infection with blood-borne diseases and staff must take care. Staff are advised to use disposable gloves to protect themselves from blood contamination when carrying out finger-prick glucose tests but this does not prevent finger-stick injury. Common causes are using the wrong lancet for that particular finger-pricking device, incorrect procedure for removing the used lancet from the device, attempting to resheath the lancet, and careless disposal of the used lancet. Never resheath a used lancet, always drop it into a sharps container immediately. Glucolet II is a device which retracts the needle into a safety cover after pricking the finger, precluding staff injury.

Strips and Meters

The first blood glucose strips, Dextrostix, were revolutionary in their day. However, they were inconvenient to use because the blood had to be washed off the strip before the result could be read. Nowadays, most people use meters. Keep them clean, handle them gently, follow the instructions, and calibrate new packs of strips. Ask the company trainer to visit the surgery each year to update staff. Use test solutions provided and share in any district quality assurance scheme for meters. Many patients buy meters off the shelf. Check they are using them properly; some are easier to use than others. Some download to computers. (See *Balance*, British Diabetic Association, February 2000.) New systems include a watch-line device which measures transcutaneous glucose using a tiny electric current; an implantable sensor which records multiple interstitial fluid glucose levels over three days; and an infrared device which transmits computerized readings over a modem. All these devices must be calibrated with finger-prick glucose levels and there are still concerns about reliability. They are all expensive.

When to test

Test whenever you want to know the blood glucose. Patients should understand that home blood-glucose monitoring allows them to check their glucose at any time, virtually anywhere, to ensure that they are safe and comfortable, and that any changes in treatment, eating, or exercise can be made on a day-to-day basis. On most occasions when a health care professional sees someone with diabetes it is sensible to measure the finger-prick blood glucose. Previously many diabetes clinics sent patients for laboratory blood glucose tests when they arrived in clinic. The patients then sat for hours while the sample was processed. Nowadays, the doctor or nurse can check the blood glucose while talking with the patient. Interestingly, when the old system of having a lab glucose, then waiting for the result was abolished in our clinic, some patients thought they had not had a 'proper check-up' despite having finger-prick glucose and a glycosylated haemoglobin estimation.

Professionals Should test patients at least once a year, and preferably during every visit to the clinic. Test ill patients at least four times a day.

Insulin-treated patients Should test before each meal and before bed until their blood glucose levels are stable. Patients using short-acting insulin pens or pumps should continue to test four times a day for optimum flexibility in insulin dosage adjustment and glucose control. If the number of tests is being reduced, the one which should always remain is the pre-bedtime test to ensure that patients go to bed with a safe glucose concentration.

Non-insulin-treated patients Can test three or four times a day when treatment has just started or if their treatment regimen has been changed. The most important test for those with Type 2 diabetes is the pre-breakfast, fasting test as this is a useful indicator of overall glucose balance and it should ideally be 4–6 mmol/l. These patients can learn how to adjust their tablets according to blood glucose levels.

Illness, pregnancy, or exercise More frequent finger-prick glucose tests may be needed in illness or pregnancy, or when undergoing new, hazardous, or vigorous exercise.

Glycosylated haemoglobin

Many proteins are glycosylated, that is, bound with glucose. Haemoglobin A1$_c$ (HbA1$_c$) is the one which is most often used to monitor glucose balance. HbA1$_c$ is related to the concentrations of glucose in the blood over the half life of the red cell, about 6 to 8 weeks. There are several different methods for measuring glycosylated haemoglobin, those measuring total HbA1 being less sensitive than those measuring $HbA1_c$ itself. This means that each laboratory's normal range will differ. A level above 10 per cent of total haemoglobin is always too high.

$HbA1_c$ will be affected by anything which alters the rate of production or destruction of red cells and by the presence of abnormal haemoglobins e.g. HbF. It is also affected by frequent transfusions.

$HbA1_c$ looks at the past, but has the advantage of being an average indication of blood glucose concentration. A finger-prick blood glucose relates to now, and has the disadvantage of being merely one of many changes in concentration during an average day.

Glycosylated haemoglobin should be measured at least once a year, and preferably on every visit more than two months since the last test. Patients can attend the laboratory for an estimation a week or two before being seen in clinic so that the result is available for discussion. Some units estimate this in blood-spots on filter paper or little finger-prick collector bottles sent in by the patient a week or two in advance.

Some centres use fructosamine which measures glycosylation of several plasma proteins, especially albumin. It therefore reflects glucose balance one or two weeks before the sample is taken. Fructosamine is affected by anything which influences plasma protein levels and should be corrected for plasma protein level. It is not regarded as such a reliable test as $HbA1_c$ but is quicker and cheaper to measure, and does reflect a shorter time span.

Summary

♦ Hyperglycaemia is one manifestation of diabetes which is a multisystem disorder.

♦ The laboratory venous glucose is the only criterion for formal diagnosis of diabetes. Laboratory glucose levels should be checked from time to time in patients in whom other glycaemic monitoring techniques are in use.

♦ For everyday use, finger-prick blood glucose monitoring provides instant assessment of blood glucose concentration any time, anywhere. It can be used by professionals and patients or their carers.

♦ Finger-prick blood glucose testing is a laboratory method carried out away from the laboratory. The results are only of use if the test is performed accurately, according to instructions.

♦ Pay attention to each stage of the testing technique, whether performed by doctor, nurse, or patient.

♦ People with abnormal colour vision must not use visually read strips without a meter.

♦ All meters and sensors must be used according to instructions: the result is only as good as the user's technique.

- Anyone with diabetes can use finger-prick blood glucose measurement providing they can understand what they are doing and why and are properly taught with regular revision sessions.
- Finger-prick blood glucose testing is more useful than urine glucose testing.
- Glycosylated protein estimation, usually haemoglobin $A1_c$ percentage, represents longer-term blood glucose concentration. This should be performed at least once a year, and preferably more often.

Chapter 8

Oral hypoglycaemic treatment

Who should take oral hypoglycaemic drugs?

Consider oral hypoglycaemic drugs for patients whose blood glucose control is poor despite dietary effort (see Table 8.1), and who do not require insulin injections. Set individual targets for blood glucose or glycosylated haemoglobin taking the patient's overall clinical and mental state, and home circumstances into consideration. A strict glucose balance is not always appropriate in a very elderly person living alone, for example. Oral hypoglycaemic agents work only if the patient has some residual insulin production. They should be avoided in patients with Type 1 diabetes for whom insulin treatment is essential.

Which drug?

The drugs used are a biguanide (metformin), sulphonylureas (e.g. glibenclamide, gliclazide, glimepiride), thiazolidinediones (rosiglitazone, pioglitazone), prandial glucose regulators (repaglinide, nateglinide), a alpha-glucosidase inhibitor (acarbose), and a high-fibre product (guar gum). Metformin and glibenclamide (and glipizide in fewer patients) were used in UKPDS-(see p. 29). None of the other agents has had such lengthy study in so many patients.

Table 8.1 Target blood glucose concentrations in people with diabetes

	Blood glucose level (mmol/l)
Fasting	4.0–6.0
Random	4.0–7.0
Haemoglobin A1$_c$ (%)	*Laboratory normal range

Set targets according to each individual's age, general health, and circumstances. Avoid hypoglycaemia.

Note: Non-diabetics and diabetic patients on diet alone may have blood glucose levels below 4.0 mmol/l under normal circumstances—hypoglycaemia is not diagnosed until the blood glucose is below 2.2 mmol/l. However, in patients taking glucose-lowering drugs or insulin it is safest to keep the blood glucose above 4.0 mmol/l.

* Laboratory normal range will vary. DCCT-aligned laboratories—target <7 per cent.

Metformin

Metformin reduces appetite. Glucose absorption from the gut is reduced and glucose uptake into tissues is enhanced. Metformin's effects are predominantly upon the glucose rise after a meal. Pancreatic insulin production is not enhanced by metformin. It lowers the blood glucose towards normal but is unlikely to cause hypoglycaemia. Metformin also has a lipid-lowering effect. It is often given in combination with sulphonylureas.

Consider metformin as the initial treatment for:

1 *Obese patients* because metformin may reduce appetite and may be less likely to cause weight gain than sulphonylureas.

2 *Vocational drivers*—of large goods vehicles, passenger-carrying vehicles, and trains should be started on metformin because of the minimal risk of hypoglycaemia.

3 *Those who operate hazardous machinery, or others in whom hypoglycaemia would be especially dangerous.*

4 *Older patients*—consider metformin because of the reduced risk of hypoglycaemia—but beware the risk of lactic acidosis in those with cardiac, renal, or hepatic disease.

All patients should understand that these tablets are to help correct a permanent fault in the pancreas—too little insulin released at the wrong time. Some patients assume they are taking a course of pills, like antibiotics, or think that a few taken intermittently will suffice. It is also the prescriber's responsibility to ensure that people with diabetes are fully informed about their medication and its potential hazards.

The usual dosage range is 500–1700 mg a day in divided doses after meals. However, some physicians prescribe up to 2000 mg daily, and a few prescribe 3000 mg daily suggesting that this increase may enhance the weight-reducing effect even though glucose balance is normal. It is important to start gently and to encourage the patient to give the drug at least a month's trial if possible as some patients who experience side-effects develop tolerance.

Side-effects

Gastrointestinal effects are common and include loss of appetite, a metallic taste in the mouth, nausea, vomiting, flatulence, abdominal cramping, and diarrhoea. Vitamin B_{12} and folate deficiency may occur in people on big doses for a long time. Lactic acidosis is a rare but potentially fatal side-effect which should be avoided by careful selection of patients. It is most commonly seen in elderly people with renal impairment or in patients with hepatic impairment or alcohol excess.

Tests

Measure vitamin B_{12} levels annually in patients on 1500 mg or more a day, and measure plasma creatinine annually in patients without renal impairment, and at least six-monthly in those with impairment. If the creatinine rises stop the metformin and discuss the patient's treatment with a diabetologist.

Table 8.2 Information for patients on metformin

1. Your diabetes tablets are called metformin.
   Take . . . . . mg (. . . tablet) with or after breakfast;
   Take . . . . . mg (. . . tablet) with or after lunch;
   Take . . . . . mg (. . . tablet) with or after main evening meal.

2. Metformin will help your diabetes diet to control your blood glucose level. It will only help you to lose weight if you stick to a weight-reducing diet.

3. The tablets will work only if you take them regularly as prescribed!

4. If you are too unwell to take your tablets for any reason contact your doctor or diabetes nurse immediately.

5. If you cannot eat, or are vomiting, do not take your tablets but contact your doctor or diabetes nurse immediately.

6. Occasionally metformin can cause stomach and bowel upsets but these are often temporary and less likely if treatment is started gradually. Never exceed your alcohol limit (ask your doctor what this should be)—excess alcohol could make you extremely ill. Large doses of metformin may cause anaemia by reducing vitamin B_{12} and folate absorption so people taking 1500 g or more a day should have an annual blood count and their vitamin B_{12} level checked. Patients with severe kidney trouble should not take metformin. Ensure your doctor checks your kidney function regularly.

7. Over the years your diabetes may slowly progress. As your pancreas 'wears out' the tablets may become less effective. Some people may need insulin injections eventually. You may also need insulin temporarily if you are ill or have an operation.

8. Although your diabetes does not need insulin treatment at present you must take just as much care of yourself in general as someone on insulin injections. There is no such thing as mild diabetes. Your doctor will help you to stay well.

9. Carry a diabetes card with you.

This table may be photocopied for use by patients only. © 2002 Dr Rowan Hillson. From *Practical diabetes care*, Oxford University Press, 2002.

Contraindications and cautions

The contraindications for metformin include: pregnancy and breast feeding; alcoholism; renal, hepatic, and cardiac failure; severe infection; trauma; dehydration; ketoacidosis. Cimetidine reduces renal clearance of metformin. The dose of warfarin may need adjusting.

Sulphonylureas

The drugs, their dosage and approximate duration of action are shown in Table 8.3. Start with a small dose which can be increased every few days according to blood glucose concentrations. Increase chlorpropamide at weekly intervals or longer because of its long half-life.

Side-effects

Hypoglycaemia may occur. All sulphonylureas can cause allergic rashes, gastrointestinal disturbances (usually mild) such as anorexia, nausea, and vomiting, and, rarely, reduction in platelets, white cells, or aplastic anaemia. They can also cause flushing with alcohol although this is particularly pronounced with chlorpropamide. Weight gain may be a problem in some patients. Cholestatic jaundice (usually reversible) may occur with chlorpropamide and hepatic dysfunction may be caused by some sulphonylureas. Chlorpropamide also has an anti-diuretic hormone-like action and hyponatraemia is not uncommon, especially in people taking diuretics.

Contraindications and cautions

Diabetic ketoacidosis, pregnancy, and breast-feeding. Caution in renal or hepatic dysfunction. Various drug interactions with sulphonylureas are outlined in Table 8.5.

Which sulphonylurea?

The one you are used to. Chlorpropamide is taken once daily and can provide gentle action because it is so long-acting. However, it can cause prolonged hypoglycaemia and may be dangerous in the elderly. Glibenclamide is widely used. It is much longer-acting than people think. The glucose-lowering effect may last over 24 hours, especially in renal impairment. Glibenclamide enters the pancreatic islets. It may cause profound

Table 8.3 Sulphonylureas

Name	Dosage range per 24 hrs	Dosage frequency
Chlorpropamide	50–500 mg	once a day
Gliclazide	40–320 mg	once/twice a day
Gliclazide as Diamicron 30 MR	30–120 mg	once a day
Glimepiride	1–6 mg	once a day
Glipizide	2.5–20 mg	once/twice a day
Gliquidone	15–180 mg	one to three times a day
Tolbutamide	500–2000 mg	one to three times a day

Table 8.4 Information for patients on sulphonylurea tablets

1. Your diabetes tablets are called . . . .
They belong to a family of medicines called sulphonylureas.
Take . . . . mg (. . . . . tablet(s)) before breakfast;
Take . . . . mg (. . . . . tablet(s)) before main evening meal.

2. The tablets will help your diabetic diet to control your blood glucose level.

3. The tablets will work only if you take them regularly as prescribed!

4. If you are too unwell to take your tablets for any reason contact your doctor or diabetes nurse immediately.

5. If you cannot eat, or are vomiting, do not take your tablets but contact your doctor or diabetes nurse immediately.

6. Side-effects are usually mild and infrequent and include stomach or bowel upset and headache. Flushing may occur with alcohol. Allergic rashes, jaundice, and blood problems occur rarely.

7. These tablets work by reducing the blood glucose. Sometimes the blood glucose may fall too low (i.e. below 4 mmol/l). This is called hypogly-caemia and may happen if you are taking too big a dose, eat too little, or exercise more than you expect. If you feel muddled, slow-thinking, tingly, unduly emotional or cross, sweaty, shaky or notice your heart thumping fast, eat some glucose, then have a big snack. Contact your doctor or diabetes nurse. You may need to reduce your dose of tablets.

8. Over the years your diabetes may slowly progress. As your pancreas 'wears out' the tablets may become less effective. Some people may need insulin injections eventually. You may also need insulin temporarily if you are ill or have an operation.

9. Although your diabetes does not need insulin treatment at present you must take just as much care of yourself in general as someone on insulin injections. There is no such thing as mild diabetes. Your doctor will help you to stay well.

10. Always carry a diabetes card and some glucose with you.

Table 8.5 Drug interactions with sulphonylureas

	Lower blood glucose	Raise blood glucose
General	Alcohol (+flushing)	
Antimicrobials	Chloramphenicol Co-trimoxazole Miconazole Sulphonamides	Rifampicin
Cardiovascular	Beta blockers (+reduce hypo warning)	Diazoxide Loop diuretics (Nifedipine) Thiazides
Anticoagulant	Warfarin	
Gastrointestinal	H2 antagonists	
Endocrine/Metabolic	Octreotide	Corticosteroids Contraceptives
Joints	Aspirin Phenylbutazone NSAIDs Sulphinpyrazone Azapropazone	
Psychotropic	MAOIs	Lithium Phenobarbitone Tricyclics (+postural hypotension)

hypoglycaemia on as small a dose as 2.5 mg and can also cause prolonged hypoglycaemia. Glibenclamide is the commonest cause of hypoglycaemia due to oral agents. One in three patients taking glibenclamide experience hypoglycaemia. Tolbutamide and glipizide are both short-acting and can be linked to meals to allow some patients flexibility in dosage—small meals, small dose; big meal, big dose. Gliclazide reduces platelet stickiness which could reduce the risk of vascular complications, but glucose-lowering itself can have effects on platelets. Gliclazide also seems less likely to produce sudden hypoglycaemia than glibenclamide; it is becoming increasingly popular but costs more.

At risk patients

1 *Old age* Start on a very small dose and increase it cautiously. Tolbutamide or glipizide are short-acting and perhaps safer. Gliclazide may also be used but is longer-acting. Emphasize the need for regular meals.

2 *Cardiac disease* Metformin may cause lactic acidosis in severe cardiac failure or hypotension. With sulphonylureas beta blockers can reduce symptoms of hypoglycaemia and thiazide diuretics reduce the glucose-lowering effect. ACE inhibitors may cause hypoglycaemia.

3 *Renal disease* All glucose-lowering agents are potentially hazardous in patients with reduced creatinine clearance. Gliclazide and gliquidone are the best options but insulin will probably be needed. Metformin is contra-indicated in severe renal impairment.

4 *Hepatic disease* The liver is involved in the metabolism and/or excretion of all sulphonylureas, so these are usually avoided. Metformin is also contraindicated as lactic acid accumulation can occur in hepatic decompensation. Alcohol excess can predispose to lactic acidosis. This means that patients with severe hepatic disease should be insulin-treated (and in an alcoholic, for example, this can be difficult).

5 *Gastrointestinal disease* Any condition which should seriously impair absorption of oral medication is an indication for insulin therapy. Cimetidine interacts with both metformin and sulphonylureas.

6 *Arthritis* Anti-inflammatory drugs, including aspirin can also potentiate the hypoglycaemic effect of sulphonylureas in various ways.

7 *Anti-coagulant treatment* May displace sulphonylureas from protein binding and potentiate their action, and vice versa.

8 *Allergy to sulphonamides* Precludes the use of sulphonylureas.

9 *Porphyria* Do not give sulphonylureas.

Combined therapy

If patients on sulphonylureas or metformin fail to achieve acceptable blood glucose levels, add the other agent. The combination of a sulphonylurea and metformin produces significant glucose lowering and may stave off insulin therapy for some years. Some doctors give small doses of each together early in treatment because each potentiates the action of the other.

In UKPDS (34): 'When metformin was prescribed in the trial in both non-overweight and overweight patients already treated with sulphonylurea there was a significant increase in the risk of diabetes-related death and all-cause mortality.' The authors point out that the patients on sulphonylurea were older, more hyperglycaemic, and followed up for five years less. They concluded: 'The epidemiological analysis did not corroborate an association of diabetes-related deaths with combined sulphonylurea and metformin therapy although the confidence intervals were wide.' The National Institute for Clinical Excellence (NICE) in its *Guidance on rosiglitazone* states 'Patients with inadequate blood glucose control on oral monotherapy (metformin or sulphonylurea) should first be offered metformin and sulphonylurea combination therapy, unless there are contraindications or tolerability problems.'

Thiazolidinediones

These drugs are peroxisome proliferator-activated receptor-gamma (PPAR-gamma) agonists and work by reducing the body's resistance to insulin action. Rosiglitazone is the subject of a technology appraisal by NICE (NICE 2000). It is currently licensed for use

> in oral combination treatment of Type 2 diabetes mellitus in patients with insufficient glycaemic control despite maximal tolerated dose of oral monotherapy with either metformin or a sulphonylurea:
>
> > in combination with metformin only in obese patients.
> >
> > in combination with a sulphonylurea only in patients who show intolerance to metformin or for whom metformin is contraindicated.

NICE also points out that if patients have persistent blood glucose elevation on either metformin or sulphonylurea they should be offered a combination of those two agents. Only if this combination fails to control blood glucose levels or cannot be tolerated should they be offered rosiglitazone as above. It is better to combine rosiglitazone with metformin than with a sulphonylurea. Rosiglitazone should NOT be added to combined metformin *and* sulphonylurea. The indications for pioglitazone are similar to those of rosiglitazone.

Side-effects

Hypoglycaemia may occur. Hyperlipidaemia (increased LDL and HDL cholesterol), anaemia (thought to be due to haemodilution), and oedema are well-recognized. Cardiac failure may be precipitated or worsened, although this seems primarily to occur if these agents are used in combination with insulin (the combination is contraindicated). Weight gain, headache, gastrointestinal symptoms, abnormal vision, arthralgia, dizziness, fatigue, and lactic acidosis may also occur. Women with polycystic ovary syndrome may ovulate as insulin resistance is reduced. Troglitazone, the first thiazolidinedione on the UK market, was withdrawn because of reports of liver damage. Rosiglitazone and pioglitazone may cause hepatic dysfunction and should be stopped if liver enzymes are more than three times the upper limit of normal.

Contraindications and cautions

Check liver function, renal function, full blood count, and lipids before prescribing. Do not prescribe thiazolidinediones if there is evidence of liver impairment, severe renal dysfunction (creatinine clearance below 4 mls/min), or cardiac failure. Monitor lipids regularly, and liver function every two months. It would seem sensible to monitor full blood count too. The manufacturers advise stopping the drugs if ALT is over three times the upper limit of normal. Thiazolidinediones should not be combined with insulin and are contraindicated in women planning pregnancy, during pregnancy, or whilst breast-feeding.

Prandial glucose regulators

Like sulphonylureas, these drugs act by increasing insulin release from the pancreas. The main advantage is rapid absorption and action which means they can be taken before meals—whenever they are. Because of the short duration of action these agents are unlikely to cause hypoglycaemia, and may be particularly helpful in patients who suffer fasting hypoglycaemia on sulphonylureas. They may be combined with metformin, but not with other glucose-lowering drugs (and nateglinide cannot at present be used as monotherapy). Repaglinide is usually started with a dose of 0.5 mg within 15 minutes before each main meal. If transferring from another glucose-lowering drug you will probably need to start with 1 mg of repaglinide before each main meal. The dose is titrated every one to two weeks according to finger-prick blood glucose measurements. Nateglinide is started in patients whose glucose is not controlled on metformin alone, usually with 60 mg, 1 to 30 minutes before breakfast, lunch, and evening meal.

Prandial glucose regulators are probably the most flexible glucose-lowering tablets and may allow sophisticated glucose management by patients who wish this. However, there may be compliance problems as these drugs must be taken with each main meal.

Side-effects

Hypoglycaemia can occur (glucose will stimulate further insulin release so continue monitoring, and further glucose and food as necessary for six hours). Other side-effects include visual disturbances, gastrointestinal symptoms, rash, and transient elevation in liver enzymes. It would seem prudent to stop the drug if liver enzymes rise over three times the upper limit of normal.

Contraindications

These include severe renal or hepatic impairment, pregnancy, and lactation.

Interactions

Repaglinide may interact with MAOIs, beta-blockers, ACE inhibitors, salicylates, non-steroidal anti-inflammatory drugs, octreotide, alcohol, anabolic steroids, oral contraceptives, thiazide diuretics, corticosteroids, thyroid hormones, sympathomimetics, rifampicin, and simvastatin. The list for nateglinide includes ACE inhibitors and drugs which inhibit cytochrome P450.

Monitoring of oral hypoglycaemic therapy

1 *Patient knowledge* Does the patient know what and how much he is taking? What is it for? What should he do if he becomes ill? What precautions should he take? Is he aware of potential side-effects? Is the patient on sulphonylureas aware of the risk and symptoms of hypoglycaemia?

2 *Diabetes card?* Ask the patient to show it to you.

3 *Carrying glucose?* Ask to see it.

4 *Hypoglycaemia* Have patients on sulphonylureas experienced this?

5 *Blood glucose balance* If the blood glucose is persistently above your targets for that patient despite maximal oral therapy, the patient usually needs insulin.

6 *Clinical state* Apart from usual tissue damage monitoring, have any conditions arisen which make it inadvisable to continue oral hypoglycaemics? Is there any evidence of side-effects of treatment?

7 *Laboratory monitoring* Consider checking electrolytes (hyponatraemia), creatinine clearance (risk of hypoglycaemia or lactic acidosis), full blood count (folate or B_{12} deficiency), liver function. Check B_{12} annually in metformin-treated patients (taking ≥ 1500 mg).

8 *Take home message* Write down the dose the patient should be taking and when.

Sick days and missed tablets

If the patient misses a tablet he should not take double next time! Discuss each case individually. If the error is realized within two hours of the correct time take the missed dose immediately. In someone on once daily breakfast-time therapy, the missed dose could be taken within four hours of the correct time. If the patient has a vomiting illness or severe diarrhoea not only will he be unable to keep his tablets down (or fail to absorb them) but the illness is likely to push his blood glucose concentration up. The patient must contact his doctor immediately. Monitor the blood glucose carefully and use insulin to control it. Keep a particularly careful eye on elderly patients' blood glucose levels—vague confusion may indicate hypoglycaemia. Non-specific symptoms can be accompanied by gross metabolic derangement and high glucose levels.

Guar gum

This polysaccharide increases gastric transit time, slows carbohydrate absorption, hence lowering postprandial blood glucose rise; it also sequesters bile acids. It may reduce LDL cholesterol. It can be used in Type 1 or Type 2 patients to improve blood glucose balance. Its use around the UK is variable.

The dose is one 5 g sachet with each meal either sprinkled over the food or stirred into it. The meal must be accompanied by at least 100 ml water or water-based drink. Alternatively it can be stirred into a drink (e.g. half glass of fruit juice) and drunk immediately before the meal. It is advisable to start with a smaller dose at first (see packet insert).

It should not be given to patients with swallowing problems or oesophageal disease and should be used with caution in those with other gastrointestinal disorders. It may slow the absorption of other drugs which should be taken an hour before the guar gum.

Patients on sulphonylureas or insulin must be warned that they may experience hypoglycaemia as their blood glucose levels fall.

Side-effects are usually gastrointestinal—flatulence and diarrhoea. The patient should maintain a good fluid intake while on guar gum.

Acarbose

This is an alpha-glucosidase inhibitor which reduces the rate of sucrose digestion in the small intestine so less glucose is absorbed after a carbohydrate meal. It is still finding its place in the treatment of diabetes in the UK.

It is used if either diet alone or other oral hypoglycaemic drugs do not lower the blood glucose to within the target range. If used on its own it will not cause hypogly-caemia. The dose is 50 mg three times a day either chewed with the first mouthful of the meal, or before food with a drink of water. Some doctors advise lower starting doses to accustomize the patient to its gastrointestinal effects. The dose can be increased after six to eight weeks to 100 mg three times a day if necessary. Larger doses should be used with care (see data sheet).

Do not give acarbose to those with gastrointestinal disorders including hernias, children under 12 years, nursing mothers, or those with renal disease.

Gastrointestinal side-effects are common. Because acarbose interferes with carbo-hydrate metabolism, fermentation is increased and this can cause bloating, flatulence, and diarrhoea. The symptoms are worse if patients eat sugar.

If acarbose is given to patients on sulphonylureas they must be warned:

(a) that they may experience hypoglycaemia as their blood glucose levels fall;
(b) to treat hypoglycaemia with glucose not sucrose as the latter will not be digested.

Summary

♦ Oral hypoglycaemics should be used if dietary control fails.

♦ They work only if the patient is making some of their own insulin.

♦ Eventually some patients taking oral hypoglycaemic agents will need insulin.

♦ Use the drug you are most familiar with, but consider the patient and his/her needs.

♦ Oral hypoglycaemic drugs can cause hypoglycaemia—be alert for this—the symp-toms may be less clear cut than in insulin-treated patients.

♦ Patient education about therapy is as important as in insulin treatment.

♦ Tablet-treated diabetes is not mild—it can still maim, blind, or kill.

References and further reading

ABPI *Compendium of Data Sheets and Summaries of Product Characteristics 1999–2000*. Datapharm Publications Limited, 12 Whitehall, London SW1A 2DY.

eMIMS—*www.emims.net*

National Institute for Clinical Excellence (NICE) (2000). *Guidance on rosiglitazone for Type 2 diabetes mellitus*. Technology Appraisal Guidance No. 9. *www.nice.org.uk*

UK Prospective Diabetes Study Group (UKPDSG) (1998). Effect of intensive blood-glucose control with metformin on complications in overweight patients with Type 2 diabetes (UKPDS 34). *Lancet*, **352**, 854–65.

Chapter 9

Insulin treatment

'I won't have to inject insulin, will I?'

For many people, having diabetes means insulin injections. From the moment they learn that they have diabetes their thoughts may be occupied by the terror of having to inject themselves. They think that these injections will start on their first visit to the diabetic clinic. Sometimes this unexpressed anxiety can impede communication. This may be an unfounded fear, but unfortunately some people do need insulin, and, at present, this has to be given by injection.

Who needs insulin?

- All with Type 1 diabetes—such patients will die without insulin treatment.
- Those with severe symptoms of hyperglycaemia
- Those with acute onset of symptoms

Intense thirst and polyuria can be devastating (p. 3). Insulin always cures these symptoms by reliably reducing the blood glucose towards normal. Thus all such patients should be considered for insulin therapy, at least initially, to make them feel better. If the symptoms have arisen within weeks or have progressed rapidly it is likely that the patient requires long-term insulin therapy. If these symptoms are combined with ketosis and weight loss insulin is mandatory (Table 9.1).

Table 9.1 Target blood glucose concentrations in people with Type 1 diabetes

	Target finger-prick whole blood glucose level (mmol/l)
Before meals	4.0–7.0
Before bed	6.0–8.0*
Haemoglobin A1$_c$ % †	4.5–6.4

Set targets according to each individual's age, general health, and circumstances. Strict glucose balance is not always appropriate in a very elderly person living alone, for example. Take care to avoid hypoglycaemia and always reduce the blood glucose gradually.
* This is to reduce the risk of nocturnal hypoglycaemia and assumes that bedtime is 4–6 hours after the last meal. Patients on insulin should always have a bedtime snack.
† This will vary according to the laboratory's upper limit of normal, In DCCT (p. 29) the mean HbA1$_c$ of the intensively treated group which showed such a dramatic reduction in tissue damage, was 7 per cent.

Ketone-producers

In someone with diabetes who is not on a strict weight-reducing diet and whose blood glucose concentration is in double figures (i.e. 10 mmol/l or more), moderate to large ketonuria indicates the need for insulin therapy.

Insulin treatment is life-saving in acute diabetic ketoacidosis. Any patient who has had an episode of proven diabetic ketoacidosis in the past is likely to need lifelong insulin treatment. Rarely, patients subsequently produce enough of their own insulin to return to oral hypoglycaemic therapy. However, they should be encouraged to test their blood glucose particularly assiduously during intercurrent illness or stress. They should keep insulin in the refrigerator for immediate use if the blood glucose concentration rises so that a further episode of ketoacidosis can be averted.

People who have lost weight unintentionally

Marked weight loss in anyone with newly diagnosed diabetes may indicate the need for insulin treatment. This is especially likely in people who have lost weight despite eating well. It is difficult to define 'marked weight loss' but that in excess of 3 kg (half a stone) should be viewed seriously.

Ill people

People with diabetes who have an infection, a myocardial infarct, an accident, or a surgical illness often need insulin until the additional illness is under control. The necessity of insulin treatment should be assessed in all diabetics urgently admitted to hospital.

Children and young people

The majority of people whose diabetes develops under the age of 30 years have Type 1 diabetes with an absolute insulin requirement. In this group the decision **not** to use insulin should be taken very carefully.

Pregnant women

It is usual to give insulin to pregnant women with diabetes who cannot control their blood glucose by diet alone.

Patients hyperglycaemic despite oral hypoglycaemic drugs

Patients whose random blood glucose tests are usually above 8 mmol/l, fasting 6 mmol/l, or who have a persistently raised haemoglobin $A1_c$ should be assessed as likely to benefit from insulin treatment. In obese people or those who eat a lot of sugar it may be possible to improve matters by re-evaluation of the diet.

> Delilah is 48 and has had diabetes for 14 years. Other family members in Jamaica suffer from diabetes. She has been taking maximal doses of oral hypoglycaemic drugs for some time. For the past two years her glycosylated haemoglobin has been between 15 and 20 per cent, she has lost over 10 kg in weight and has constant thirst and polyuria. Her last clinic glucose was 26.5 mmol/l. Her daughter and a succession of staff in the diabetic clinic have been attempting to persuade her to accept insulin treatment. She has had one insulin injection and said it did not hurt. But she still refuses regular insulin.

James, in his 50s, with a responsible job, also rejected insulin. His home blood glucose tests ranged from 13 to 22 mmol/l. He was constantly tired and had frequent minor infections. He felt he was not performing well at work. He accepted that his symptoms were due to persistently high blood glucose levels but refused to exchange his tablets for insulin. It transpired that he was very frightened of needles. After watching his doctor stick an insulin needle into their own leg he plucked up the courage to do the same. 'It doesn't hurt' he said, astonished. He is now taking twice daily insulin and constantly reiterates how well he feels.

Patients with complicated diabetes

Insulin has been used in patients with severe painful diabetic neuropathy, even if their glycaemic balance approximates to normal on oral therapy. The rationale is that aggressive normalization of the blood glucose with insulin may relieve the symptoms. Patients with other tissue damage may benefit.

Patients with severe hypertriglyceridaemia (i.e. 10 mmol/l or more) and diabetes may need very good control and therefore are usually treated with insulin to achieve normoglycaemia and normotriglyceridaemia. A very low fat diet and carefully balanced carbohydrate intake are needed, and lipid-lowering drugs may also be required (p. 137).

Insulin species

There are many insulin preparations on the market (Table 9.2). Despite this variety, there are only two main insulin manufacturers marketing insulin in the United Kingdom— Novo Nordisk and Lilly, but CP Pharmaceuticals also market beef and human insulin.

Human insulin

This is prepared by three methods. Eli Lilly were the first company to use genetic engineering to produce a drug on a large scale. A segment of the DNA of non-pathogenic bacteria (*Escherichia coli*) is replaced by that coding for the human proinsulin gene. The bacteria are then cultured in vats. As they multiply they produce human proinsulin. The bacteria are destroyed and the proinsulin is converted to insulin, purified, and marketed as the range of Humulin insulins (prb insulin). Novo Nordisk manipulate the genetic material of a yeast in a similar manner to produce pyr insulin. Previously they modified pork insulin using an enzyme reaction—enzymatically modified pork or emp insulin. Prb insulins and pyr insulins are suitable for strict vegetarians or those whose religious beliefs proscribe ingestion of pork or beef. Emp insulin cannot be used in this way.

It was hoped that human insulin would be less antigenic than animal insulins. This is not entirely so—antibodies are found in patients taking human insulin.

Human insulin and hypoglycaemia

In recent years there has been concern that human insulin use may be associated with reduced warning of hypoglycaemia. Several careful studies have shown that this is not so. However, the whole matter highlighted the need to consider the effects of recent care improvements on the daily lives of our patients, and on the incidence of hypoglycaemia.

Table 9.2 Insulin preparation available in the UK

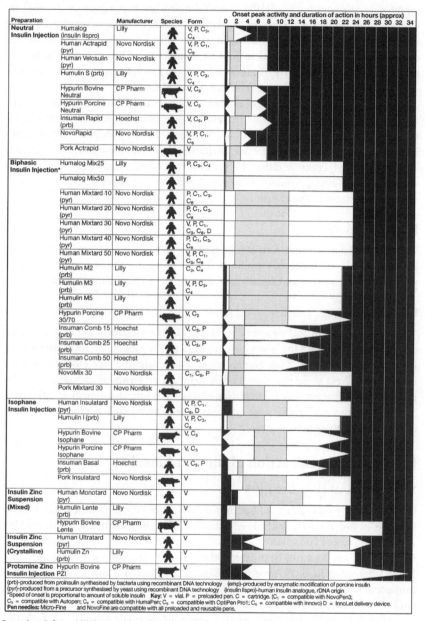

Preparation		Manufacturer	Species	Form	Onset peak activity and duration of action in hours (approx) 0 2 4 6 8 10 12 14 16 18 20 22 24 26 28 30 32 34
Neutral Insulin Injection	Humalog (insulin lispro)	Lilly		V, P, C₃, C₄	
	Human Actrapid (pyr)	Novo Nordisk		V, P, C₁, C₆	
	Human Velosulin (pyr)	Novo Nordisk		V	
	Humulin S (prb)	Lilly		V, P, C₃, C₄	
	Hypurin Bovine Neutral	CP Pharm		V, C₃	
	Hypurin Porcine Neutral	CP Pharm		V, C₃	
	Insuman Rapid (prb)	Hoechst		V, C₅, P	
	NovoRapid	Novo Nordisk		V, P, C₁, C₆	
	Pork Actrapid	Novo Nordisk		V	
Biphasic Insulin Injection*	Humalog Mix25	Lilly		P, C₃, C₄	
	Humalog Mix50	Lilly		P	
	Human Mixtard 10 (pyr)	Novo Nordisk		P, C₁, C₃, C₆	
	Human Mixtard 20 (pyr)	Novo Nordisk		P, C₁, C₃, C₆	
	Human Mixtard 30 (pyr)	Novo Nordisk		V, P, C₁, C₃, C₆, D	
	Human Mixtard 40 (pyr)	Novo Nordisk		P, C₁, C₃, C₆	
	Human Mixtard 50 (pyr)	Novo Nordisk		V, P, C₁, C₃, C₆	
	Humulin M2 (prb)	Lilly		C₃, C₄	
	Humulin M3 (prb)	Lilly		V, P, C₃, C₄	
	Humulin M5 (prb)	Lilly		V	
	Hypurin Porcine 30/70	CP Pharm		V, C₃	
	Insuman Comb 15 (prb)	Hoechst		V, C₅, P	
	Insuman Comb 25 (prb)	Hoechst		V, C₅, P	
	Insuman Comb 50 (prb)	Hoechst		V, C₅, P	
	NovoMix 30	Novo Nordisk		C₁, C₆, P	
	Pork Mixtard 30	Novo Nordisk		V	
Isophane Insulin Injection	Human Insulatard (pyr)	Novo Nordisk		V, P, C₁, C₆, D	
	Humulin I (prb)	Lilly		V, P, C₃, C₄	
	Hypurin Bovine Isophane	CP Pharm		V, C₃	
	Hypurin Porcine Isophane	CP Pharm		V, C₃	
	Insuman Basal (prb)	Hoechst		V, C₅, P	
	Pork Insulatard	Novo Nordisk		V	
Insulin Zinc Suspension (Mixed)	Human Monotard (pyr)	Novo Nordisk		V	
	Humulin Lente (prb)	Lilly		V	
	Hypurin Bovine Lente	CP Pharm		V	
Insulin Zinc Suspension (Crystalline)	Human Ultratard (pyr)	Novo Nordisk		V	
	Humulin Zn (prb)	Lilly		V	
Protamine Zinc Insulin Injection PZI	Hypurin Bovine	CP Pharm		V	

(prb)-produced from proinsulin synthesised by bacteria using recombinant DNA technology (emp)-produced by enzymatic modification of porcine insulin
(pyr)-produced from a precursor synthesised by yeast using recombinant DNA technology (insulin lispro)-human insulin analogue, rDNA origin
*Speed of onset is proportional to amount of soluble insulin **Key:** V = vial. P = preloaded pen. C = cartridge. (C₁ = compatible with NovoPen3;
C₃ = compatible with Autopen; C₄ = compatible with HumaPen; C₅ = compatible with OptiPen Pro1; C₆ = compatible with Innovo) D = InnoLet delivery device.
Pen needles: Micro-Fine   and NovoFine are compatible with all preloaded and reusable pens.

Reproduced from MIMS *Monthly Index of Medical Specialities* with permission. This table is updated monthly; please see the current issue for up-to-date information.

Highly purified insulin is less antigenic than older insulins so small dose changes may have a larger glucose-lowering effect than that of an older insulin in a long-term user. Near-normoglycaemia means an increased risk of hypoglycaemia with fewer warning symptoms. The concentrated U100 insulin requires more precision in drawing up than, say, the obsolete, U20 insulin. It seems likely that all these factors played a role in the development of hypoglycaemia in people with long-standing insulin-treated diabetes coincidentally changed to human insulin. In addition, long duration of diabetes may be associated with reduction in warning symptoms of hypoglycaemia.

There are still some patients who believe that they have better warning of hypoglycaemia on animal insulin than on human insulin. Animal insulins are still readily available and these patients should be kept on their preferred insulin. After all, it is the patient who is receiving the insulin, not their doctor! Whenever any patient's insulin is changed, whatever the make or species, they must be warned that they may experience hypoglycaemia at different times than they would usually expect and perhaps with different warning symptoms. Always listen to your patients. Their treatment must be acceptable to them.

Porcine insulin

This is obtained from pig pancreas. It is one amino acid different from human insulin and was widely used. Porcine insulin is slightly antigenic although modern highly purified insulins rarely cause clinically noticeable problems through antibody formation.

Beef insulin

This is obtained from beef pancreas. It is still available for patients who wish to continue taking it, although the larger insulin producers no longer market it. Beef insulin is a little more antigenic than human or porcine insulin, but the older forms were much more likely to produce antibodies than newer forms. High antibody levels mean that the patient needs increasing doses of insulin to remain in glycaemic balance, until uncomfortably large amounts have to be injected. Antibody formation is also linked with insulin fat atrophy.

Duration and peak action of different insulins

Very short-acting insulins

These insulins are modified so that they do not form hexamers which take time to separate. Active insulin is available straightaway. They are absorbed and start working within 15 minutes of injection and clear in two to five hours. Very rapidly acting insulins can (and indeed must) be injected either immediately before eating, or during or immediately after food. Better glucose balance is achieved if the insulin is injected immediately before food. However, if one is uncertain what food will be provided (in a restaurant, for example) insulin can be injected as the meal finishes.

Insulin lispro (Humalog) and Insulin aspart (Novorapid) can be used in basal–bolus insulin patterns, or mixed with intermediate-acting insulins in twice daily regimens. Because insulin levels peak with the glucose absorption from food they produce an insulin effect close to that of the normal pancreas. Because the insulin more closely matches the food, proper use of such insulins reduces the frequency of hypoglycaemia. However, hypoglycaemia can occur, and it may come on quickly and be severe. The other problem can be that the insulin 'runs out' before the next injection and meal. Thus there can be postprandial normoglycaemia or hypoglycaemia, but preprandial hyperglycaemia.

Very short-acting insulins are increasingly popular with patients as they allow more flexibility of lifestyle and enable patients more scope for fine-tuning their glucose than older insulins. Some patients use ultra-short-acting insulins for some meals and short-acting insulins for others. This produces a very complex pattern and is only suitable for patients who are very knowledgeable and careful about diabetes self care.

Short-acting insulin

The insulin made by the normal human pancreas is a clear, colourless fluid which, when released into the bloodstream via the portal vein, produces an effect upon the blood glucose within minutes. All short-acting insulins are clear and colourless. They include Actrapid, Velosulin, Insuman Rapid, Hypurin Porcine, or Bovine Neutral and Humulin S (R in USA). The main difference between insulin in the non-diabetic and insulin in the diabetic person is its route of delivery into the bloodstream and the lack of fine control. There is a tendency to forget that the effect of human insulin released by the pancreas in direct response to circulating blood glucose concentrations cannot be the same as the effect of subcutaneous insulin absorbed regardless of the blood glucose concentration. Even continuous intravenous insulin infusion cannot mimic the finely tuned response of the normal pancreas.

Intermediate-acting and long-acting insulins

These cloudy insulin suspensions are modified to reduce their solubility and hence to prolong their absorption from the insulin injection site. There are several methods of modifying insulins. A newer basal insulin, glargine, is clear. It cannot be mixed with other insulins.

Isophane (NPH) insulin is produced by adding protamine and a small amount of zinc at the body's normal pH. This produces insulins which last for about 12 hours. Examples of isophane (NPH) insulins are Humulin I, Insuman Basal, Hypurin Bovine, Porcine Isophane, and Insulatard g.e.. Short-acting insulin can be mixed with isophane insulins and the mixture will remain stable. This is the basis of the fixed proportion mixtures, or of mixtures made by the patient themselves.

Zinc is used to precipitate insulin crystals, hence the insulin zinc suspensions. Insulin is absorbed slowly into the bloodstream from these crystals in the injection site. These insulins are Lente, Semilente, and Ultralente: current versions include Monotard, Semitard, Humulin ZN, and Ultratard. Mixtures of these insulins with short-acting insulin are not stable.

Protamine zinc insulin (PZI) has more protamine and zinc than isophane insulin. This prolongs the action of the insulin.

Combination or pre-mixed insulins

Also available are stable mixtures containing varying proportions of short-acting insulin and isophane (NPH) insulin. There are mixtures containing as little as 10 per cent or as much as 50 per cent short-acting insulin. These mixtures are inflexible—if the dose is increased, both the short-acting and the isophane insulin dose is increased. However, they have gained in popularity because of their simplicity and their avoidance of drawing-up errors (pp. 87, 88). Names include the Mixtard range (10 to 50), Humulin M2, Humalog Mix 25, Insuman Comb range, Pork Mixtard 30.

Concentration of insulin

All insulin in the United Kingdom is provided as 100 units per millilitre. Other countries do not all conform to this system and patients should be very careful if they obtain their insulin abroad.

Insulin in the users' hands

While manufacturers and pharmacists keep insulin in appropriate conditions (at 4–10 °C during storage) people with diabetes and their carers may be less careful. Teach them how to look after their insulin properly.

The insulin in a bottle is usable if it has been kept at temperatures between 4 and 25 °C, is within its expiry date, has a properly sealed bung, has not been contaminated (e.g. clear insulin contaminated with cloudy), has been mixed gently if a cloudy insulin (but not been shaken into foam), and is the right insulin for that person at that injection time.

If the patient places a suspension insulin in an over-cold refrigerator or too close to the ice compartment it may freeze and the insulin crystals may degrade. If insulin vials are kept near a radiator, or in a hot car, or simply on a shelf in a very hot country the insulin will gradually clump as the protein is cooked (like egg white). Exposure to light will also cause insulin degradation. All vials so treated will have reduced potency and raised antigenicity.

The commonest form of contamination is the introduction of cloudy insulin into the clear bottle by the uneducated self-mixer who has forgotten that one should draw up the clear insulin first (see p. 88). Another form of contamination is to leave short-acting insulin and zinc suspension insulins in the syringe for more than a few seconds before injection. The short-acting insulin will gradually be converted to slower acting insulin. Bacteria can be introduced during drawing-up but the preservative should kill them. Other contaminants may be introduced from the syringe. People who draw up insulin and flush it vigorously in and out of the syringe and the insulin bottle to clear air bubbles may shear off microscopic amounts of plastic from the syringe which is then introduced into the insulin. This may lead to complaints that the syringe sticks (because of friction between the plunger and minute scratches inside the syringe). Re-education is required.

Modified insulins, the longer-acting insulins, should be mixed gently by rotating the bottle between the two hands before drawing-up the dose, or the amount of insulin complex injected may vary. Over-zealous mixing can make the insulin foam and this causes frustrating delay in clearing air bubbles and measuring the right dose.

It may sound naïve to point out that the patient or their carer should give the right insulin for that person for that occasion. Mistakes happen all too easily.

> Jeremiah had had diabetes for over 50 years. He continued to mix his own soluble and isophane insulins. He had frequent, severe hypoglycaemia. Eventually a young registrar discovered that for over 50 years Jeremiah had believed that his clear insulin was slow-acting and his cloudy insulin worked quickly. No young whipper-snapper of a hospital doctor was going to convince him otherwise. However, he had survived many years of diabetes despite this basic misconception.

Insulin injection equipment

The basic equipment

A syringe and needle. There are several U100 insulin syringes on the market. Half-millilitre syringes can contain up to 50 units of insulin; one-millilitre syringes, 100 units of insulin. There are also 0.3-millilitre syringes.

Most syringes have integral needles which are very fine and well-lubricated, causing minimal trauma at injection. The potential problem with such fine bore needles is sticking with some cloudy insulins, but this is rarely a problem. They bend easily and if inserted up to the hilt and bent there is possibility of the needle snapping and remaining *in situ*. This is very uncommon in practice. These needles have revolution-ized the previously unpleasant task of self-injection. It can now be described, truthfully, as 'no more than a gnat bite'.

Insulin pen devices

These devices have an insulin cartridge instead of ink and a double-ended needle instead of a nib. This pierces the bung of the insulin cartridge ready for use. The insulin dose is dialled up or clicked in at the other end of the pen. A plunger pushes the bottom of the cartridge down, ejecting the chosen dose of insulin through the needle.

Each device has a slightly different action. The pen does the same job as a syringe and needle but there is no need to draw up the insulin dose from a bottle. This improves accuracy although with the models in which the patient has to depress the plunger repeatedly to administer the insulin it is possible to lose count. Insulin pens are also much more portable than a full syringe and needle and can be carried in a pocket or bag without the insulin in the cartridge 'going off'.

Choose the best pen for each user. Different pens have different features including: the way in which the insulin dose is selected, whether this is counted or dialled up, the ease of operation, delivery of the dose (either by a twisting motion or depressing a plunger), knowing whether the insulin has gone in, knowing how much insulin is left, and when to change the cartridge. Most devices are quite robust. There are chunky pens which are easy to grip, those with concealed needles, and one which delivers 0.5 units of insulin charges. It is essential to teach the patient how to prime the pen, load an insulin cart-ridge, and how to expel air from the needle before each injection. Patients are usually advised to hold the pen vertically, needle up, and waste a few units of insulin before each injection to clear the needle of air. If there is air in the needle or cartridge this may

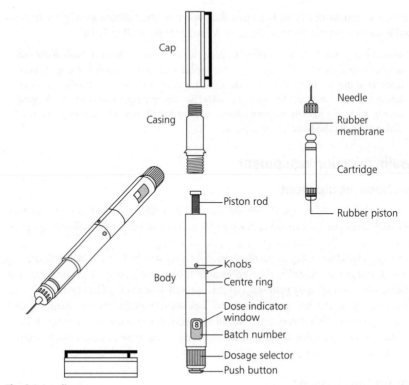

Fig. 9.1 Insulin pen

remain undetected and cause dosage errors. The patient must always read the instructions and practise with a diabetes specialist nurse or other person trained in pen use.

There is now a range of pre-loaded disposable insulin pens. Virtually all the patient has to do is screw on a pen-needle, dial up the dose, and inject the insulin. Loading errors are abolished as the insulin is already in the pen. These pens can be used for patients of all ages, including some elderly people or their families who might otherwise need supervision by the district nurse. These pens cannot deliver a dose smaller than two units which may be difficult for patients on small doses. Pre-loaded, disposable pens currently available on prescription include Actrapid, Insulatard, Mixtard (10, 20, 30, 40, 50), and Novorapid (Novo Nordisk) and the Lilly Humaject range.

Single units of insulin can be given with the Autopen, BD pen Ultra, Humapen, Innovo, and Novopen 3 devices. Half units can be injected with Novopen 3 Demi. Magnifiers are available for people with poor vision. Insulins available for pen injection are updated from time to time (check the *Monthly Index of Medical Specialities*—MIMS). They include Actrapid, Humalog, Humulin S, Hypurin Bovine or Porcine Neutral, Insuman Rapid, Novorapid; Humulin I, Hypurin Bovine or Porcine Insulatard, Insulatard; Humalog Mix25, Humulin M2, Insuman Comb (15, 25), Mixtard (10, 20, 30, 40, 50).

All patients on insulin should be considered for insulin pen therapy—it is usually more accurate, convenient, comfortable, and practical. But it is the patient who must choose the method he or she prefers.

Continuous subcutaneous insulin (CSII) pumps

CSII has been available for about 20 years. Many specialist centres tried it initially but problems with pumps and the hazards of ketoacidosis, combined with the widespread use of insulin pens in basal bolus regimens, slowed the more general introduction of CSII. Nowadays, about 0.1 per cent of insulin-treated patients in the UK use CSII, compared with 5 per cent in the USA and some other European countries. Newer, safer pumps are now being reintroduced to the UK.

CSII is not a method for a non-specialist centre. It needs full 24-hour back-up from people who are very familiar with the technique. The danger is of diabetic ketoacidosis if insulin delivery is interrupted. This method needs considerable commitment from patient and staff. Diabetes UK, in their position statement in August 2000, advises that people most suited to pump therapy

> must have a good knowledge and understanding of diabetes; be well motivated and willing to take control of their diabetes; be prepared to test blood glucose levels at least four times a day and be confident in acting on those results; have an awareness of how insulin, exercise and food intake affect blood glucose levels.

Implantable insulin infusion devices

There have been several implantable insulin pumps with an insulin reservoir which can be filled through the skin. The insulin is pumped either directly into a vein or intraperitoneally. At present they are mainly used as a last resort in people in whom no other method has succeeded in preventing frequent diabetic ketoacidosis. When reliable implantable glucose sensors are widely available there will be further exciting possibilities with implantable systems—the aim being to have a fully automated system which measures the glucose, calculates the insulin dose, and gives it.

Insulin jet injectors

These 'guns' drive insulin spray through the skin. They are sometimes used in the USA but rarely in Britain. They may help people with needle phobia but can leave lumps, bruises, or sore areas at the injection site and insulin may ooze out afterwards. Needle-phobic patients are usually better with devices which hide the needle from view.

Other methods of giving insulin

Oral insulin is not feasible without some means of protecting the insulin from digestion. Recently capsules which release their insulin into the colon have been tried. Other studies enveloped oral insulin in lipid globules to be absorbed in their entirety and then enzymatically processed in the blood stream. Intranasal insulin has been used experimentally and is partially effective but absorption may be altered by nasal problems.

Re-use of disposable equipment

All needles, lancets, and syringes are pre-packed and sterilized by the manufacturers. They are made for single use only.

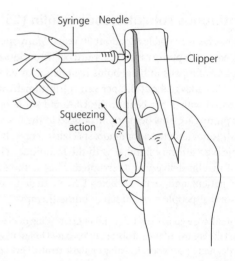

Fig. 9.2 Needle clippers in use

Disposal of sharps and syringes

It is each professional's and patient's personal responsibility to ensure that used sharps and used syringes are properly disposed of. Every patient should have a needle clipper (B-D Safeclip and others) and use it. The clipped and thus unusable syringes can then be put in a sharps box to be returned to the chemist, hospital, or surgery for formal disposal. Professionals must be aware of the potential for needle-stick injuries when clipping needles, emptying finger-pricking devices, and handling lancets. Needles and lancets should never be resheathed.

Administering insulin

Drawing up insulin

Drawing insulin into a syringe to the correct dose with no air requires dexterity, concentration, good vision, and a steady hand. The bottle of insulin should be in date and the top should be clean (to clean use 70 per cent alcohol). Bottles of cloudy insulin should be rotated gently between two hands to mix the insulin. The insulin bottle is held vertically bung-down and the needle is inserted vertically so that insulin, not air, is drawn up. It is easier to withdraw insulin if air is injected into the bottle first. Air in the syringe can be expelled by tapping or by re-injecting insulin into the bottle to expel air bubbles. The dose is then checked and the needle withdrawn from the bung.

If insulins are to be mixed in the syringe it is important that the clear, short-acting insulin is not contaminated with cloudy, slower-acting insulin. Therefore the clear insulin is drawn up first. However, once the clear insulin has been drawn up the correct dose of cloudy insulin and **no more** must be drawn up. This technique is fraught with error. Some advisers suggest drawing up each insulin separately and injecting each through a detachable needle left in the skin or completely separately. Isophane

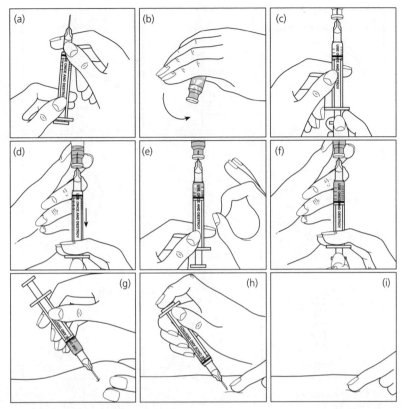

(a) Attach needle to syringe if necessary
(b) Gently rotate bottle to mix insulin
(c) Draw up air and inject into the insulin bottle
(d) Draw up insulin
(e) Clear air bubbles
(f) Check syringe contains correct insulin dose
(g) Inject insulin into fatty layer under skin
(h) Withdraw needle
(i) Press on the hole

Fig. 9.3 Drawing up and injecting insulin

(NPH) insulins make stable mixtures with short-acting insulins, but all the others are not stable and should be injected immediately.

Injecting insulin

Insulin is injected subcutaneously. If the injection is too shallow, a painful intradermal blister may be raised. Insulin absorption will be unpredictable. If the injection is too deep the insulin will enter the muscles where it will be absorbed more rapidly than anticipated. It is important that patients understand what is meant by subcutaneous. It is not enough to say 'under the skin'. The patient should take a thick pinch of skin

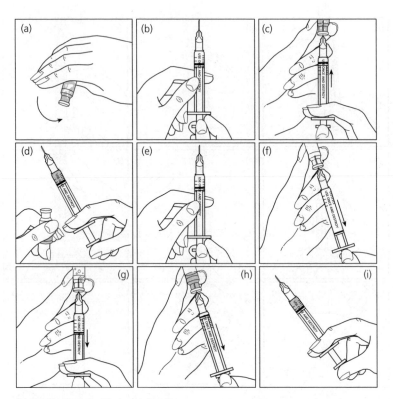

(a) Gently rotate bottle to mix insulin
(b) Draw up air
(c) Inject air into cloudy insulin bottle
(d) Put cloudy insulin down
(e) Draw up air
(f) Inject air into clear insulin bottle. Draw up clear insulin
(g) Express air bubbles and check you have drawn up correct dose of
     clear insulin
(h) Draw up correct dose of cloudy insulin
(i) Ready for injection

Fig. 9.4 Mixing insulin

and subcutaneous tissue and insert the needle at an angle of 45°. The insulin is then injected, the needle left *in situ* for a few seconds, and then withdrawn. Some patients press a clean tissue, cotton wool swab, or finger over the hole for a few moments.

If the skin is dirty it should be washed and dried. There is no need to use alcohol or other spirit swabs unless the person cannot wash. These may cause the injection to sting and surgical spirit hardens the skin. Bruising occurs occasionally as does a tiny trickle of blood. Patients need to be reassured that this is most unlikely to mean that the insulin has been injected intravenously. Some doctors advocate withdrawing the plunger before injection to ensure that a vein has not been entered, but many no longer consider this useful.

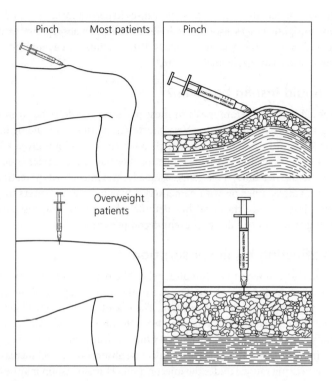

Fig. 9.5 Injecting insulin

Insulin injection sites

The most commonly used sites are the thighs, upper buttocks, abdomen, and upper arms. A few patients use their calves and forearms. The conventional wisdom is that patients should rotate their injection sites e.g. left arm Monday morning, left abdomen Monday evening, left thigh Tuesday morning, right thigh Tuesday evening, etc. This is to avoid overuse of a particular site. However, insulin absorption varies with each injection site. It is most rapid from the abdomen, then the arms, thighs, and buttocks. A multi-site rotation scheme can therefore cause variability in blood glucose balance although this may be more of a problem in some people than others. It may be better to use, say the abdomen during the day and thighs at night, or to use the left and right side of a particular site for a week or two and then change. Patients who are prepared to monitor this closely with blood-glucose testing can work out which site is most appropriate for which circumstance.

Patients will all have favourite sites, usually those which are easy to reach, and there will be areas which gradually become numb through repeated use. Occasionally one discovers small black holes in a patient's leg or abdomen into which he or she has been putting insulin for years.

Insulin has a direct effect on fat cells and causes hypertrophy at overused injection sites. These unsightly bulges also cause variability in insulin absorption. Atrophy due to insulin antibodies is rarely seen nowadays. Patients must be encouraged to use the whole extent of each available injection site.

When should insulin be given?

Insulin should be given before meals in most patients. The delay between injection and eating is usually 10–30 minutes. Very short-acting insulins should be injected as the patient sits down to eat—or immediately afterwards. Insulin is given after meals more often than we realize—patients forget, or they have never understood when to give it, or the district nurse is late. Occasionally in someone whose eating is very erratic (for example, a person with dementia) it may be safer for carers to give very short-acting insulin once the meal has definitely been eaten and just give a little longer-acting insulin once a day to prevent decompensation.

Factors affecting insulin absorption

These are myriad and tend to be forgotten when the patient and diabetes adviser are poring over the blood glucose diary. The size of the insulin depot and the amount of fat surrounding the depot affects absorption. The rate of entry into the blood stream is determined by the circulation through and from the injection site. Thus cold or other stimuli causing vasoconstriction such as nicotine or drugs will reduce absorption, as will shock from whatever cause. Heat will increase absorption as will increased blood flow to an exercising muscle under the injection site. Human insulin may be absorbed more rapidly than porcine insulin.

> A student came home and put his supper on to cook. He injected his insulin then had a warm bath. He was found in the water unconscious from hypoglycaemia. Fortunately his head had not submerged.

The amount of insulin cleared within 24 hours from an injection site can vary from 20 to 100 per cent from person to person and within the same person. With such considerable variability in insulin absorption added to the effects of food, exercise, and emotion, the mystery is not why the blood glucose balance is so variable, but why it is possible to control it at all!

Common insulin regimens

Once daily long-acting insulin ± short-acting insulin

This regimen was popular some years ago and remains popular with patients as it requires only one injection a day. However, it rarely produces good glucose control unless the patient is making some of their own insulin. Situations in which it can be useful are as an adjuvant to oral hypoglycaemic therapy; when a carer such as a district nurse has to come in to give the insulin to someone who cannot inject their own; or in someone in whom the aim of treatment is not normoglycaemia but freedom from symptoms and avoidance of hypoglycaemia or marked hyperglycaemia. This regimen is not appropriate for the majority of patients.

The insulins used are usually Monotard or Ultratard, often with a short-acting insulin mixed and injected immediately.

Twice daily injections of a fixed proportion mixture

This regimen was previously viewed with horror by some diabetologists as it has little flexibility. However, now that a larger range of mixtures is available patients can have a 30:70 mixture before breakfast and a 10:90 mixture before their evening meal, for example. Patients find it simple and convenient and drawing-up errors are minimized. It is probably the easiest regimen to start with and can be converted to a more flexible pattern if required. Fixed proportion mixtures are often used for children with diabetes. For many people the 30:70 mix appears to provide near normoglycaemia. Insulin pens can deliver mixtures (see p. 79).

Twice daily short-acting and longer-acting insulin

This is a very flexible and popular regimen. The usual insulins are a short-acting such as Actrapid or Humulin S and an isophane such as Insulatard g.e. or Humulin I, or a porcine or human lente insulin such as Monotard. This regimen gives four points at which the insulin dose can be adjusted. It is essential that the patient understands this—many do not have a clear idea of when their insulins act (like Jeremiah, p. 83) and make inappropriate adjustments. Full use of this regimen is possible only with knowledgeable home blood glucose monitoring.

> Joan was pregnant and was trying hard to maintain normoglycaemia. She was on twice daily Actrapid and Monotard insulin. She was troubled by nocturnal and pre-breakfast hypoglycaemia so she reduced her morning Actrapid insulin. She should have reduced her evening Monotard.

Thrice daily short-acting insulin and once daily longer-acting insulin

This provides sophisticated and flexible insulin treatment which can often allow a very varied lifestyle. The principle is to provide background insulin overnight using isophane (NPH) or Ultratard insulin, and to give short-acting insulin before each meal. Sometimes twice daily isophane is needed. The dose of short-acting insulin is adjusted according to blood glucose at that time, food to be eaten, and activity planned. The insulin is usually given with a pen injector (see p. 83). Nowadays, many patients prefer very short-acting insulin before meals (see p. 80). Properly used both this regimen and the preceding one can produce normoglycaemia. However, to do so requires a sophisticated use of insulin sliding scales and careful observation by the patient of their glucose responses to insulin, food, and activity. The use of thrice daily insulin does not, in itself, produce better glucose control.

This regimen is very popular with patients and many find that they can move meals and even omit them. Others, however, still need regular mealtimes and snacks, and all must eat a bedtime snack to guard against nocturnal hypoglycaemia.

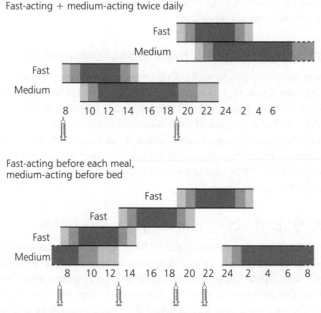

Fig. 9.6 Insulin injection regimens. Dark shading = maximum glucose-lowering effect. The onset, intensity, and duration of insulin action varies from person to person day to day. Insulin action and duration is shorter with very short-acting insulins

Monitoring of people on insulin therapy

It is the patient who injects the insulin, not the doctor

The doctor prescribing the insulin is not the person who has to inject it and live with what happens thereafter. The insulin regimen must be tailored to the needs of the each person with diabetes. If the patient cannot control their blood glucose on a particular regimen, finds it hard to use, or loses confidence in it, it should be changed. Clearly, it is worth giving each new regimen a few months' proper trial with full education and continued support. If a patient moves to your clinic from elsewhere on a bizarre insulin regimen which seems totally illogical but appears to satisfy them, do not change it until you have had a chance to assess how it works for that person.

1 *Patient knowledge*

(a) *Theory* Does the patient know which insulins and how much of each he is taking? What is the insulin for? When is each insulin likely to act? Does he know how to adjust the dose according to blood glucose levels, diet, and activity? What should he do if he becomes ill? What precautions should he take? Is he aware of the risk and symptoms of hypoglycaemia?

(b) *Practical* Does the patient know how to check, store, and draw up his insulin? Does he know how to inject it? Does he know what to do with unused and used sharps and syringes? Have you watched him draw up and inject insulin? Does he know how to use his insulin pen, including changing cartridges? Have you watched him do this?

Table 9.3 Information for patients on insulin injections

1. Insulin name   Dose injected before: breakfast/lunch/evening meal/bed

   . . . .

   . . . .

   . . . .

2. Your insulin type is human/porcine/beef.

3. Inject your insulin using a syringe/pen.

4. Inject your insulin subcutaneously—this means into the fatty tissue under the skin of the thighs, abdomen, buttocks, or upper arms.

5. Inject your pre-meal insulin . . . . minutes before food. Eat three meals a day with mid-morning, mid-afternoon and pre-bed snack unless otherwise advised.

6. Insulin lowers the blood glucose level and will help to control your blood glucose level.

7. Sometimes the blood glucose may fall too low (i.e. below 4 mmol/1). This is called hypoglycaemia and may happen if you are taking too big a dose, eat too little or exercise more than you expect. If you feel muddled, slow-thinking, tingly, unduly emotional or cross, sweaty, shaky, or notice your heart thumping fast, eat some glucose, then have a big snack. Contact your doctor or diabetes nurse. You may need to reduce your dose of insulin.

8. Insulin will work only if you inject it regularly as prescribed!

9. If you are unable to take your insulin for any reason contact your doctor or diabetic nurse immediately.

10. Never stop your insulin. If you cannot eat, or are vomiting, contact your doctor immediately or follow the sick day rules he has given you.

11. Always carry a diabetic card and some glucose with you.

This table may be photocopied for use by patients only. © Dr Rowan Hillson, 2002. From *Practical diabetes care*, Oxford University Press, 2002.

2 *Diabetes card*? Ask the patient to show it to you.

3 *Carrying glucose*? Ask to see it.

4 *Glucagon* Has the patient's partner or relative an up-to-date supply and does he/she know how to use it? (See p. 101)

5 *Hypoglycaemia* Has the patient experienced this? Does he have warning symptoms? Does he have nocturnal hypoglycaemia?

6 *Blood glucose balance* (Table 9.1) If the blood glucose is persistently outside your targets for that patient, the patient's treatment needs adjusting.

7 *Clinical state* Apart from usual tissue damage monitoring, have any conditions arisen which would alter the insulin regimen? Is there any evidence of side-effects of treatment? Have you examined the injection sites?

8 *Laboratory monitoring* Consider checking renal function as this will alter insulin clearance.

9 *Driving* Has the patient told the DVLA he is on insulin? Does he know how to drive safely on insulin?

10 *Take home message* What does should the patient be taking now? When should it be taken? Write it down.

Remember that the patient knows his or her diabetes far better than you do. Listen to their observations carefully and do not contradict them without due thought. For example, they are usually right in their belief that the pharmacist has given them the wrong insulin—this happens occasionally. They are usually correct in saying that a particular insulin does not suit them. And even if they do harbour misconceptions, correct them gently with an appropriate explanation.

The whole principle of insulin treatment is that the insulin is adjusted to the patient's lifestyle and not the other way around. People should not have to eat to keep up with their insulin—lower the dose to suit what they want to eat. People should not be prevented from doing particular things because they have to go home and inject their insulin—give them an insulin pen to carry with them. They should not be afraid that hypoglycaemia will ruin their work or a day out. Learn about your patient as a person and fit the diabetes treatment around his or her needs.

Summary

+ If the patient needs insulin prescribe it—the sooner the better.

+ Choose the insulin regimen that suits the patient's needs.

+ An insulin regimen will succeed only if the person using it understands how their insulin(s) work and can adjust it according to insulin need.

+ Remember the factors influencing insulin absorption from the injection site.

+ Choose the equipment appropriate to the patient's needs and keep up to date with advances in insulin delivery.

Chapter 10

A low blood glucose—hypoglycaemia

Some patients may feel that health care professionals are more concerned about normalization of blood glucose concentration than the occasional hypoglycaemic episode. But for the person who has diabetes, hypoglycaemia can be a terrifying experience to be avoided at all costs. To this end the person may aim for persistent hyperglycaemia, preferring the absence of hypoglycaemia now to the vague and distant threat of long-term tissue damage. Many older patients still cling to the old advice to 'keep a little sugar in your urine'. The professionals who are most likely to brush aside anxieties about hypoglycaemia are those who have never experienced it themselves, or have, so far, not encountered a hypoglycaemic patient who has had an accident or caused one.

The price of normoglycaemia is often hypoglycaemia. Doctors should watch that their zealous quest for a normal glucose to reduce the likelihood of tissue damage does not create problems for their patients.

> Joseph always kept his blood glucose between 4 and 6 mmol/l by careful control of his diet and his insulin. He went on an outdoor activity course. Like everyone else unaccustomed to outdoor activities he was given detailed advice to eat more and to reduce his insulin to avoid hypoglycaemia. He agreed. On day 1 he was hypoglycaemic while climbing. He was told to reduce his insulin further and the dietitian reiterated advice to eat more at mealtimes and snacks. Next day he lost consciousness and had to be revived with glucose. The group then revealed that Joseph had been leaving his food at meal times, and had been seen throwing his snack away. Joseph subsequently admitted that he had not reduced his insulin at all. When asked why, he said that his doctor had told him he would go blind if his glucose went above 6 mmol/l.

Approximately a third of people with insulin-treated diabetes will experience hypoglycaemic coma; 2–3 per cent of insulin-treated patients have frequent severe hypoglycaemia.

Hypoglycaemia used to be considered rare in sulphonylurea-treated patients but with the current focus on normoglycaemia this is no longer the case: about a third of patients on glibenclamide experience hypoglycaemia. Patients taking metformin alone are rarely at risk of hypoglycaemia unless the metformin is taken in overdose.

What is hypoglycaemia?

'When I feel my glucose is low'

For a person with diabetes, hypoglycaemia usually means 'when I feel that my glucose is low and I don't expect it to be'. Some patients discount symptoms before meals, or

Table 10.1 Common symptoms of hypoglycaemia

Sweating	Weakness
Trembling	Hunger
Inability to concentrate	Blurred vision

Any person with diabetes treated with glucose-lowering medication who behaves oddly in any way whatsoever is hypoglycaemic until proven otherwise.

(Hepburn *et al.* 1992)

with exercise—when they expect to feel a little low, and report only those episodes which have occurred at other times. Other patients discount episodes which they have succeeded in treating themselves and describe hypoglycaemia only when someone else had to revive them. Many people with diabetes are unaware of some or all their hypoglycaemic episodes. Some patients who monitor their blood glucose regularly will deny hypoglycaemia despite recording a value of 2 mmol/l or less, because, to them, the only real hypoglycaemia is that which makes them *feel* unwell. Symptoms of hypoglycaemia, described in detail below, are by definition subjective and vary from person to person and from episode to episode (Table 10.1). Symptomatic hypogly-caemia is therefore not a good way in which to define hypoglycaemia.

When counter-regulatory hormones are released

As the blood glucose falls, it stimulates release of adrenaline, noradrenaline, glucagon, cortisol, and growth hormone. Adrenaline causes tachycardia with palpitations and tremor. Glucagon released from the pancreatic islet cells stimulates glucose release from the liver. However, in people with diabetes the glucagon response may be blunted or absent and excess insulin inhibits liver glucose release. The 'emergency' hormonal response to hypoglycaemia is called counter-regulation.

Hypoglycaemia could be defined as the blood glucose level at which the body initiates its emergency response. However, this point varies according to the pre-vailing blood glucose balance in that person. In people with persistently high blood glucose levels, counter-regulation may occur at a blood glucose of 5 mmol/l or higher. This explains why some patients complain that they feel hypo at blood glucose levels not normally regarded as hypoglycaemic. In those whose blood glucose is usually nor-mal, significant counter-regulation may not occur until the glucose is under 2 mmol/l. As patients tend to rely on the autonomic symptoms to warn of hypoglycaemia, they may have little time to act before the falling glucose level incapacitates them.

Blood glucose concentration

Hypoglycaemia is usually defined as a blood glucose below 2.2 mmol/l. Most people counter-regulate in some way at these glucose concentrations. At low blood glucose levels blood glucose testing strips may be difficult to read accurately by eye. A meter is better. It is safest to tell patients that if their blood glucose is below 4 mmol/l they should stop what they are doing and eat a snack or a meal. They should check their glucose again soon. In a potentially dangerous situation or where rapid relief of symptoms of hypoglycaemia is required, they should stop and eat glucose, followed by a snack or meal, and check their blood glucose again soon (see p. 100).

Signs and symptoms of hypoglycaemia

The most frequently reported symptoms are sweating, trembling, inability to concentrate, weakness, hunger, and blurred vision (Table 10.1; Hepburn *et al.* 1992).

Changes in thinking and perceiving

Subtle changes in the ability to perform psychological tests may occur before the patient is aware that there is a problem. Altered perception includes blurred vision, *déjà vu*, distancing from the world around, colour changes (for example, everything turns pink), altered intensity of sound, or other sensation. Time appears to slow down. Time estimation is involved in assessment of speed so hypoglycaemia may cause accidents to pedestrians and car drivers.

Concentration is poor. The person has a short attention span and can easily be distracted. He may return to the same point of the task again and again. Slow decision-making is a very common feature of hypoglycaemia. Simple decisions become insoluble conundra. The person can be well aware that they should know the answer and that the problem is simple, but find themselves unable to resolve it. Conversation may not flow smoothly as it is hard for the person to work out what to say next. Once a task has been taken on, a hypoglycaemic person may not relinquish it rather like a record stuck in the same groove: 'I've started so I'll finish'. This can be dangerous, as in the hypoglycaemic driver who will not stop driving even though he realizes his blood glucose is low.

> I watched a hypoglycaemic man trying to open a sealed polythene bag to remove an apple. His sweaty hands kept slipping but for many minutes he persisted with the same unsuccessful movements, refusing to be distracted by proffered glucose tablets. Eventually, after I had pushed glucose into his mouth, he allowed me to help extract the apple.

As the blood glucose level continues to fall the person becomes increasingly confused although they are often able to articulate this as it happens: 'I'm all anyhow, tee hee!'. The confusion may be patchy—for example, the person may become hopelessly muddled with mental arithmetic and yet be capable of driving a car (but not safely).

Emotions

Hypoglycaemia is often associated with irritation and frustration. Small setbacks may induce fast-rising rage out of all proportion to the problem. Anger may be aroused by the efforts of well-meaning helpers who are then told to 'Go away and leave me alone!' Some patients may recognize the onset of hypoglycaemia by the way they feel compelled to snap at their spouse and family. They feel contrite afterwards but say 'I just can't help myself'. Others may feel unaccountably depressed and burst into tears. Alternatively, everything is wonderful, glorious, exciting, or hilariously funny. A change in personality may be an early and subtle sign. Any behaviour which is out of character may be due to hypoglycaemia.

Refusal of help

Patients commonly refuse help when hypoglycaemic. This can lead to difficult scenes, particularly if the carer is a friend or relative of the hypoglycaemic person. Independence may be fiercely guarded and help rejected. The sufferer may be convinced that he is coping well. He may also convince relatives that this is so.

> A woman with insulin-dependent diabetes became clinically and biochemically hypoglycaemic post-partum. She was very aggressive and distressed, and refused all treatment for her hypoglycaemia. Her husband, who was with her, also refused to allow medical staff to restore her glucose to normal, presumably because he failed to realize that her hypoglycaemia rendered her unable to make rational decisions. She was on a ward unused to dealing with people with diabetes.

Hunger with or without abhorrence of food

Most symptomatic hypoglycaemic people complain of hunger, and many will eat ravenously. However, food may be rejected. This abhorrence of food is a common feature of hypoglycaemia and shows the split thinking of the hypoglycaemic person. Part of the brain may recognize the hypoglycaemia and the need to eat, while another part is revolted by the food, despite intense hunger.

Panic and hyperactivity

Cerebral irritation may combine with the stirring effects of catecholamines to produce panic, terror, and the desire to flee. Carers may be perceived as pursuers. The lack of glucose for muscle energy does not prevent considerable strength or stamina and I have seen more than one hypoglycaemic person run up hill for some distance.

> A 70-year-old woman, severely hypoglycaemic and apparently drowsy, suddenly tried to hurl herself off the casualty trolley. In the ensuing struggle this little old lady injured two ambulance men, a nurse, a muscular medical student, and a doctor while they attempted to treat her hypoglycaemia.

Skin colour changes

Adrenaline causes skin pallor but flushing or blotchy rashes may also occur in hypoglycaemia.

Sweating

Some patients wait until they experience sweating before diagnosing hypoglycaemia. It may be a late phenomenon. This is sometimes more evident to the observer than to the patient, who may, at times, ignore sweat running down his face and soaking his clothes. This effect has been used in hypoglycaemia alarms which measure changes in skin resistance due to sweating and bleep to awaken a sleeping person (assuming that they are not already unconscious).

Palpitations and tachycardia

Another common symptom of hypoglycaemia is an uncomfortable awareness of the heart's action—a moderate increase in heart rate and a feeling that the heart is pounding abnormally strongly. The systolic blood pressure may rise.

Respiratory changes

Adrenaline release can cause initial apnoea but also induces hyperventilation. Some patients are uncomfortably aware of their breathing while hypoglycaemic. Cheyne—Stokes breathing may be observed, especially in comatose patients.

Tingling

Unlike the prolonged paraesthesiae of severe, recurrent spontaneous hypoglycaemia, the paraesthesiae of acute hypoglycaemia occur fleetingly, often around the mouth and lips. Paraesthesiae may also occur in the median nerve distribution in the hand, or elsewhere.

Tremor

A falling glucose level can induce a fine tremor of the hands which is not always noticeable unless sought.

Incoordination and unsteadiness

A lack of coordination may combine with sweating and tremulous hands to cause spillages and breakages. Some degree of incoordination is observable in most hypoglycaemic people but they may not always realize it themselves. Patients often describe themselves as feeling drunk and stumble readily. They may bump into others walking beside them or trip. Other patients, however, may exhibit considerable feats of balance, of which they are apparently incapable when not hypoglycaemic.

Weakness

The lack of glucose can cause a generalized muscle weakness—'as if I've run out of petrol' said one patient. Neuroglycopenia may cause limb weakness or hemiplegia, but few patients will be aware of this.

Weariness, sleep, and coma

Intense exhaustion and a compulsion to fall asleep can overwhelm the hypoglycaemic person. Increasing lassitude makes everything too much bother. There may be a gradual descent through tiredness and sleep to coma; an active, albeit muddled person may suddenly drop to the floor unconscious. People prone to the latter should not hold potentially hazardous jobs and should take especial care to avoid hypoglycaemia.

Fitting

Fitting is relatively uncommon but occurs most often with nocturnal hypoglycaemia, presumably because the early signs of a falling glucose are not perceived and acted upon by the slumbering person. It should be noted that a person who has a fit only when hypoglycaemic is not epileptic and does not usually need anticonvulsants.

No symptoms—loss of warning

Symptomless hypoglycaemia frightens people with insulin-treated diabetes. After 20 years of diabetes about 25 per cent of patients lose some or all of their warning of hypoglycaemia. Patients whose blood glucose is near normal may have reduced warning, as may patients with recurrent hypoglycaemia. Warning may be restored in some patients by raising the average blood glucose for a few weeks and by eradicating hypoglycaemia. If a patient has poor warning of hypoglycaemia they must be extremely careful to ensure that they cannot become hypoglycaemic while driving or operating machinery or performing activities in which confusion or coma could put them or others at risk.

The diagnosis of hypoglycaemia

A person on glucose-lowering treatment (whether insulin or tablets) who seems unusual or behaves oddly in any way is hypoglycaemic until proved otherwise. It is important for both patient and carers to have a high index of suspicion. This can lead to friction: one of my patients pointed out that he can no longer be angry or impatient. Any hint of this is regarded as hypoglycaemia and he is offered glucose. While he understands his family's concern he is fed up with not being allowed to express ordinary emotions.

Out and about

In a potentially hazardous situation, for example swimming or rock-climbing, the person should eat glucose immediately they suspect hypoglycaemia. Delay caused by blood testing allows the glucose to fall further with worsening of symptoms and increased risk of inappropriate behaviour or coma. Rapid recovery proves the diagnosis.

In other situations, and if the patient is capable of doing so, a finger-prick blood glucose test will confirm the diagnosis. Readings under 4 mmol/l, are taken as hypoglycaemic and treated accordingly.

Blood glucose

If the patient is severely hypoglycaemic or if there may be any diagnostic confusion or medico-legal implications, take a venous sample for laboratory blood glucose. Remember that a finger-prick glucose may be misleading. If in doubt, take blood for laboratory venous glucose and give glucose.

Sally was a psychologically-disturbed woman on insulin treatment with frequent, severe hypoglycaemia. She was admitted deeply unconscious and hypothermic having been found on a park bench. Peripheral venous access had always been a problem—there was none. She was obviously clinically hypoglycaemic. One nurse prepared a central line, another drew up some glucagon, and the third checked a finger-prick blood glucose. She put the strip into the meter and waited. '22 mmol/l', she announced. Everyone stopped and looked up in amazement. However, a repeat after the patient's finger had been washed and dried was so low that the strip did not change colour at all—less that 1 mmol/l. After glucagon and 100 ml of 50% Dextrose, Sally gradually regained consciousness and began fighting and swearing. About a year later she was found dead in the street, presumably from hypoglycaemia.

The treatment of hypoglycaemia

In patients capable of swallowing

Glucose is absorbed most rapidly in liquid form, for example Lucozade or any other glucose-containing proprietary drink. Powdered glucose can be stirred into water, juice, or milk. Glucose (dextrose) tablets are a more convenient form to carry. Glucose gel in foil packs or in polythene bottles (for example, Hypostop) is especially useful for water activities.

Follow glucose treatment with food to sustain the recovery and prevent relapse. Starchy carbohydrate, with some sugar and plenty of fibre is the most effective, such as a jam sandwich or muesli bar.

In patients who cannot, or will not swallow

Hypoglycaemic patients may irrationally reject food. This can usually be overcome by firm encouragement to eat. However, they may fight vigorously and spit out anything they are given to eat or drink. Staff should keep back to avoid personal injury and try to contain the patient in a safe area. Inject glucagon into whatever muscle bulk can be accessed safely. The alternative is to muster sufficient help to achieve venous access and inject 50 ml of 50 per cent dextrose slowly intravenously (adult dose).

Excessive hypertonic glucose can be fatal in small children. In children inject 200 mg/kg over three minutes; 50 per cent glucose contains 500 mg/ml. Thus a 25-kg (4-stone) child requires an initial injection of 5000 mg, or 10 ml, 50 per cent glucose. You can give up to 500 mg/kg in total.

Glucose is a highly irritant solution and may thrombose veins. Ensure that you are well into a large vein before injection. The best method is to insert a cannula and anchor it securely. Withdraw blood to confirm correct placement and to send to the laboratory, and inject the glucose (it is hard work because it is syrupy and two smaller syringes are easier than one big one), then flush the cannula and vein with 10–20 ml normal saline. Leave the cannula *in situ* until the person has recovered fully.

If the patient's conscious level is impaired place them in the recovery position and protect their airway. There is time to gain venous access calmly. Inject glucose intravenously, or give glucagon 0.5–1 mg intravenously or intramuscularly. Recovery is faster and more comfortable for the patient with intravenous glucose. Glucagon can cause nausea and a 'hung-over' feeling. The rise in blood glucose released by glucagon from the liver is temporary—feed the patient before they become hypoglycaemic again.

If the patient is having an epileptiform fit place them in the recovery position and safeguard them from injury. Protect the airway. Give intravenous glucose quickly. There is usually no need to give anticonvulsants as well—the convulsions will stop as the glucose rises.

After recovery check for injuries. If appropriate feed the patient or, if nil by mouth, infuse dilute intravenous glucose continuously. Elderly people tend to take longer to 'come to' after hypoglycaemia than younger ones.

Profound hypoglycaemia is rare. It is most often seen in patients who have taken deliberate insulin overdoses, in relation to alcohol, or with sulphonylureas. If 50 ml of 50 per cent glucose fails to re-establish consciousness within 15 minutes call an ambulance and give another 50 ml of glucose to adults.

What caused the hypoglycaemic episode?

Once the person is *compos mentis* again, review the sequence of events which led to the hypoglycaemic episode and derive lessons for future prevention. Often, the cause is obvious. Late for work, no breakfast, running for the train; late business meeting, missed lunch; miscalculated insulin dose; unexpected activity e.g. missed the bus, had to walk home; did not like lunch, so left it.

Patients may forget the incident entirely, so it is important to inform diabetes carers what happened.

Leo is 45 years old, and has had diabetes for 20 years. He hates coming to clinic and his response to all questions is 'I'm all right.' He denied hypoglycaemia on direct questioning. It was years before his wife, desperate for help, insisted on coming in with him to inform clinic staff that he was having frequent devastating hypoglycaemic attacks without warning. She angrily accused clinic staff of doing nothing to help her husband, and was somewhat taken aback to discover that he had repeatedly told us all was well.

Management of hypoglycaemia in insulin-treated patients

Hypoglycaemia due to excess rapid-acting insulin usually responds rapidly to glucose treatment. However, if hypoglycaemia is due to longer-acting insulin it may recur after the initial dose of oral or intravenous glucose. Ice-packs on sites of injection of large insulin overdoses may slow insulin absorption to 'buy time' for treatment.

Recurrent hypoglycaemia may be seen in patients trying to normalize their blood glucose, in people whose lifestyle or eating patterns have changed, and in various other circumstances (see Table 10.2). Recurrent, severe hypoglycaemia may be due to manipulation by psychologically-disturbed patients and can be hard to detect.

First safeguard the patient. Remove all risk of hypoglycaemia by raising the blood glucose to a constant level of about 10 mmol/l. Reduce all insulin doses by at least 25 per cent. Check insulin administration technique (from drawing up to injection, including timing—human insulin may need to be given closer to meals, even at the table). Ensure that food intake is evenly spaced throughout the day—three meals and three snacks (a pre-bed snack is vital). Test blood glucose before each meal and before bed (check technique), and sometimes during the night. Refer the patient to the hospital diabetes team urgently. Once the hypoglycaemia stops, the blood glucose will gradually be returned towards normal by gentle insulin adjustment. Sometimes such patients require hospital admission.

Table 10.2 Causes for hypoglycaemia

Common	Uncommon
Too much insulin	Autonomic neuropathy
Too much sulphonylurea	Slow gastric emptying
Too little food	Liver impairment
Exercise	Steroid insufficiency
Alcohol	Hypothyroidism
Drugs (including street drugs)	Malignancy
Renal impairment	Severe infection

Management of hypoglycaemia in sulphonylurea-treated patients

This should be regarded as similar to hypoglycaemia due to longer-acting insulin. Sulphonylureas may persist in the plasma for some time, or may continue to be absorbed from the gastrointestinal tract. This means that persisting sulphonylurea continues to stimulate insulin release from the pancreas and improve glucose uptake by the tissues, causing recurrent hypoglycaemia.

Any person with sulphonylurea-induced hypoglycaemia severe enough to require treatment from a doctor should be admitted to hospital for at least 48 hours to ensure full recovery. Patients taking glibenclamide may be hypoglycaemic for two or more days.

Causes of hypoglycaemia

Too much insulin Sometimes too much insulin is injected as a deliberate overdose. More often the dose is excessive for the patient's current needs and has been inappropriately increased by the patient or their carers. Check that the patient understands the time of maximal insulin action and its usual duration (see Table 9.2 and Fig. 9.5).

> Delia, diabetic for some years, was hypoglycaemic three times in a week, before her evening meal. She reduced her evening Mixtard insulin and increased her morning Mixtard insulin by a corresponding amount. Not surprisingly, she was severely hypoglycaemic next day. Despite her long experience with diabetes she had failed to understand that she should take preventive action by reducing her morning insulin rather than reactive action by reducing her evening insulin. She compounded the error by wrongly assuming that her total daily insulin dose must remain unchanged.
>
> An unconscious woman arrived in accident and emergency with no information. An astute house officer noted several recent injection marks in her thighs. Her finger-prick glucose was below 1 mmol/l. She was treated with intravenous glucose, and awoke after 100 ml of 50 per cent. She then admitted injecting two bottles of lente insulin. She required intravenous glucose and potassium infusion for five days and had multiple dysrhythmias despite maintaining normal electrolytes.

The insulin may arrive in the circulation earlier than expected—as from an intramuscular injection, or if the circulation to a subcutaneous site is increased (e.g. by warmth or by exercising the muscle underneath).

Too much sulphonylurea Hypoglycaemia may arise early in treatment if a new patient is started on a weight-reducing diet and oral hypoglycaemics at the same time. It can also arise if the prescriber fails to appreciate that there is considerable variation in response to oral hypoglycaemics—2.5 mg glibenclamide may render one patient severely hypoglycaemic and have no obvious effect on blood glucose in another. Always start cautiously. The medication should be given with meals. Pay attention to the recommended dosage intervals and avoid large doses in the evening. Occasionally sulphonylureas are taken in deliberate overdose by the patient, or by depressed family or friends. Never glucose-lowering drugs may also cause hypoglycaemia.

Too little food This is probably the commonest cause of hypoglycaemia. An accidentally missed meal, deliberate dieting (especially in young women), avoidance of disliked foods, missed snacks, spoiled cooking, can all contribute.

> Pierre was on a camping trip. It was his first visit to Britain and he had never tried camp cooking before. On the first night he was hypoglycaemic and required huge amounts of glucose, and other carbohydrate to maintain his blood glucose. He assured staff that he had eaten his evening meal. Next morning, despite these efforts his glucose was still low. Later that day a member of staff discovered all Pierre's food in the waste bin near the camp site. Pierre subsequently admitted that he had eaten nothing because the food had got crushed in his rucksack and he did not like to eat 'bad-looking' food.

The introduction of large amounts of fibre into the diet of someone usually on a low-fibre diet may also cause hypoglycaemia. This can occur in hospital or on diabetic holidays.

Exercise Hypoglycaemia may be caused if the person has failed to eat enough to fuel the exertion or has too much insulin in their system, preventing glucose release by the liver. Planned exercise is best coped with by reducing insulin or hypoglycaemic tablets beforehand, and, if the exercise is vigorous, by eating more. Unexpected exertion (e.g. the car running out of petrol and having to walk to a distant garage) commonly causes hypoglycaemia. The hypoglycaemia can occur at the time of the exertion and for up to 48 hours afterwards; for example, at night. This can be explained to patients as 'the body reorganizing its glucose stores after exercise.'

Alcohol People with insulin-treated diabetes who are also alcoholics run a high risk of severe, perhaps fatal, hypoglycaemia. What patients may not appreciate is that just one drink on an empty stomach may be enough to precipitate or aggravate hypoglycaemia. Every year patients find themselves guests of the constabulary who assume, at least initially, that a person who smells of alcohol and is behaving oddly, is drunk. This is one reason why every person with diabetes who is on glucose-lowering treatment should carry a diabetic card and glucose.

Drugs Beta blockers, especially non-selective ones, may reduce the warning of hypoglycaemia. Beta blockers and other hypotensive drugs as guanethidine and clonidine may reduce the response to hypoglycaemia. Some drugs potentiate the hypoglycaemic action of sulphonylureas and repaglinide—aspirin and non-steroidal anti-inflammatories, warfarin, sulphonamides, clofibrate, and fenfluramine. ACE inhibitors may cause hypoglycaemia. (See Table 8.5.)

Renal impairment Can cause severe hypoglycaemia in both insulin-treated and sulphonylurea-treated patients. If a patient has falling insulin or tablet requirements check their renal function.

> Daisy, in her 70s was admitted with severe hypoglycaemia. Her husband said that she had been having funny turns for several weeks. 'But she never missed her diabetes pills, doctor.' She had been feeling rather sick and did not fancy her food. Every morning she had been hard to awaken and had been sleepy and muddled. But her husband had woken her up to take her pills. It became clear from the history that she had had recurrent hypoglycaemia for weeks. She was found to be in renal failure.

Autonomic neuropathy May lead to delayed gastric emptying. Other factors such as pyloric obstruction can delay food digestion and absorption. Patients with severe autonomic neuropathy may have problems recognizing hypoglycaemia.

Liver impairment Can cause hypoglycaemia in a patient without diabetes. Its presence requires very careful insulin dose adjustment and frequent food intake (say every 2 hours). As most sulphonylureas and repaglinide are metabolized in the liver, they should be used with great caution in hepatic impairment, or profound hypoglycaemia will ensue. Avoid rosiglitazone and pioglitazone.

Steroid insufficiency Addison's disease should be considered in someone with inexplicable recurrent hypoglycaemia whether or not they have diabetes.

Malignancy Another cause of spontaneous hypoglycaemia in non-diabetics, but it may precipitate puzzling recurrent hypoglycaemia in people with diabetes.

Severe infection Is a rare cause of unexplained hypoglycaemia.

Hypoglycaemia and hypothermia

Hypoglycaemia and cold are a potentially lethal combination. Glucose is essential for normal thermoregulation—hypoglycaemic people cannot shiver (Gale *et al.* 1981). It is therefore essential to check a venous glucose in everyone with hypothermia, and if this is difficult, glucose should be given anyway. This particularly applies to people suffering from exposure in the mountains, at sea, or in other cold/wet/windy situations.

> An elderly diabetic woman was found on her bedroom floor. She had clearly been lying there for some time. On admission she was unconscious and had a rectal temperature of 29 °C. A finger-prick glucose would have been unreliable so a drop from a venous sample was placed on a glucose strip. It read 2 mmol/l. She was given intravenous glucose and regained consciousness. Her rectal temperature rose steadily over the next few hours with passive rewarming and she made a full recovery. It was never clear what had happened but it seemed likely that she had fallen whilst hypoglycaemic.

Never do a finger-prick blood glucose on someone with cold vasoconstricted fingers as the result, if obtained at all, will be hard to interpret. Venous blood should not be used on some glucose strips, for example, Exactech, as the results may be inaccurate.

Responsibility

Major efforts must be made to prevent hypoglycaemia. These include repeated patient and professional education. People with diabetes clearly have a choice about whether or not to accept medical advice. However, doctors and other health care professionals must ensure that patients understand that hypoglycaemia may not only cause them to injure themselves, but may cause injury to others, for example while driving a car or operating machinery, or requiring the rescue services, perhaps risking the lives of rescuers.

Carry glucose and a diabetic card

People with diabetes on glucose-lowering treatment, whether insulin or pills, should carry glucose on their person. They must be taught when to take it and replenish it once eaten. A diabetic card may help others to help them.

Summary

- Hypoglycaemia frightens patients. It may cause harm to patients or others. Prevent it.
- Hypoglycaemia is common in people taking insulin or sulphonylureas.
- Hypoglycaemia is a blood glucose below 2.2 mmol/l. For practical purposes, patients on insulin or glucose-lowering tablets with a blood glucose below 4 mmol/l should stop and eat carbohydrate. In potentially dangerous situations take glucose or bring forward a snack or meal.
- Hypoglycaemia produces many symptoms, but patients can learn to recognize their early symptoms to allow prompt treatment.
- For practical purposes, anyone with diabetes on insulin or glucose-lowering tablets who behaves oddly in any way should be assumed to be hypoglycaemic. Staff and carers should have a high index of suspicion.
- The treatment of hypoglycaemia is glucose taken either by mouth or intravenously. Glucagon should be used only if IV glucose cannot be injected.
- After treatment the cause should be sought and preventive measures instituted. Re-educate the patient (and staff if appropriate).

References and further reading

Gale, E., Bennett, T., Green, J.H., and Macdonald, I. (1981). Hypoglycaemia, hypothermia and shivering in man. *Clinical Science*, **61**, 463–9.

Hepburn, D.A., Deary, I.J., and Frier, B.M. (1992). Classification of symptoms of hypoglycaemia in insulin-treated diabetic patients using factor analysis: relation to hypoglycaemia unawareness. *Diabetic Medicine*, **9**, 70–5.

Chapter 11

High blood glucose—hyperglycaemia

One aim of the management of diabetes is to restore the blood glucose towards normal. This is not the only aim—resolution of symptoms, prevention and treatment of tissue damage, control of other metabolic imbalance, and, above all, a good quality of life are important.

Before defining hyperglycaemia, consider what blood glucose levels are desirable in each patient—the target zone. In most instances, the aim should be to maintain the blood glucose between 4 and 8 mmol/l for most of the time. The occasional random value up to 11.0 mmol/l is no worry. The fasting glucose should be below 7.0 mmol/l, ideally 4–6 mmol/l. The pre-bed blood glucose should be over 6 mmol/l in insulin-treated patients to protect them from nocturnal hypoglycaemia. (See Tables 8.1 and 9.1.)

These guidelines assume that the patient is capable of looking after themselves and not frail or vulnerable. In an elderly person with insulin-treated diabetes who lives alone it is probably better to aim for blood glucose levels between 6 and 11 mmol/l to avoid hypoglycaemia. Sometimes, for example if the patient is terminally ill, the aim is solely to avoid symptoms of uncontrolled diabetes with minimum discomfort to the patient. Tailor the target zone to the patient. Patients who keep their blood glucose under 8 mmol/l all the time may suffer from frequent hypoglycaemia.

What is hyperglycaemia?

Hyperglycaemia may be defined as the blood glucose level above the target zone for an individual patient. However, most patients have 'one-off' levels above their target zone from time to time. Action is required only if hyperglycaemia persists. This may mean for two days in a patient in whom you are aiming for strict normoglycaemia (e.g. a pregnant woman with diabetes), or for three to five days in others. It is important not to cause hypoglycaemia by overzealous normalization of the blood glucose.

Causes of hyperglycaemia

Lack of insulin A dose of insulin may be forgotten, omitted, too small, leak out of the injection site, or be poorly absorbed from the injection site. The insulin dose may be insufficient for everyday needs or insufficient because of increasing insulin demands, as in any situation when the stress hormone response is triggered (e.g. in infection). Young girls may omit or reduce insulin to cause hyperglycaemia and hence weight loss.

Lack of oral hypoglycaemic medication or failure to respond to it Some patients or their doctors do not adjust oral hypoglycaemic drugs despite persistent glycosuria or

Table 11.1 Causes of hyperglycaemia

Lack of insulin
Lack of oral hypoglycaemic medication
Failure to respond to oral hypoglycaemics
Too much food
Too little exercise
Infection
Injury—accidental or surgical
Myocardial infarction
Menstruation
Pregnancy
Emotional stress
Drugs

hyperglycaemia. Patients may forget to take their tablets. The medication may be vomited or pass through rapidly with diarrhoea. If there is inadequate insulin production in the pancreas the blood glucose will continue to rise unless insulin treatment is started.

Too much food This is a common cause of hyperglycaemia and many patients will point to occasional highs as birthday parties or treats. Christmas is usually associated with hyperglycaemia. Slim or underweight patients may need both more food and more insulin. Overweight patients should be encouraged to return to their diet.

Too little exercise Reduces energy expenditure. For example, if a previously active person changes to a sedentary job their glucose may rise.

Infection Is a common cause which should always be sought assiduously in a patient with unexplained hyperglycaemia. Insulin requirement rises rapidly with a developing infection then falls as fast as it resolves.

Injury May cause stress hormone release and increased insulin demands. Thus people with diabetes who have accidents or who undergo surgery require careful glucose monitoring.

Myocardial infarction This may be the presenting feature of diabetes especially in Asian patients. As the myocardial infarct can be silent or produce atypical symptoms, perform an ECG in any older patient with unexplained hyperglycaemia.

Menstruation May be preceded by hyperglycaemia (see p. 161) due to sex hormone fluctuations. Patients may not always volunteer this explanation of repeated hyperglycaemia.

Pregnancy Can cause unexpected hyperglycaemia in young women, whether or not they are believed to be using contraception.

Emotional stress This has unpredictable effects on the blood glucose. In theory, any stress which stimulates catecholamine release would be expected to raise the blood glucose. While hyperglycaemia is the usual response, some patients become hypoglycaemic under severe stress (e.g. fear) because of increased clearance of insulin from the injection site. Another effect of stress may be to influence the patient's management of their treatment. Anxieties about hypoglycaemia can lead to persistent hyperglycaemia. Severe psychological disturbance can be manifested by insulin omission or overdose.

Drugs Hyperglycaemia may be caused by certain drugs including steroids (e.g. in the management of asthma), thiazide diuretics, tricyclic antidepressants.

When to take action

The problem faced by all those who care for diabetes, including the people who have it, is at what blood glucose levels above the target zone to take action. If the blood glucose is over 25 mmol/l reduce it. The problem is that the blood glucose is only one factor to be considered. Consider the duration of hyperglycaemia and its cause. A one-off high glucose following a birthday party is rarely a cause for concern— although the lesson learned is to increase the amount of insulin injected before another similar party. Persistent hyperglycaemia or hyperglycaemia in an ill person needs immediate action now.

I was once asked to produce guidelines for the management of diabetic ketoacidosis for an intensive care unit. The doctor concerned wanted me to base it entirely upon blood glucose levels. I had to explain that glucose is only one facet of the metabolic derangements of ketoacidosis and that his request was impossible. Patients can have life-threatening acidosis and a blood glucose of 12 mmol/l. Other patients walk into clinic, apparently well, with a blood glucose of 30 mmol/l.

Never consider the blood glucose without assessing the patient as a whole. This will also help you to identify patients whose general condition is such that they must be managed in hospital, those who need frequent assessments as their condition might deteriorate, and those in whom there is time to adjust the blood glucose balance gradually.

Is the patient ill?

First decide if the patient appears ill or not. Then consider the degree of hyperglycaemia. Your priority is to identify patients who should be managed in hospital. Then act to control the blood glucose concentration.

Admit patients with these signs to hospital:

- altered consciousness
- confusion
- vomiting
- abdominal or chest pain
- altered respiration
- infection
- dehydration
- hypotension
- diabetic ketoacidosis

Danger signs include altered consciousness, confusion, vomiting, abdominal or chest pain, altered respiration, dehydration, and hypotension. Patients with any of these features should be seen by a doctor straightaway and admitted to hospital. Any suspicion of diabetic ketoacidosis requires immediate hospital admission. Some patients with vomiting can be managed at home (see below), but only if the doctor and the patient are experienced in diabetes care. While arranging transfer to hospital consider glucose balance. If the blood glucose is over 15 mmol/l give 4–10 units of short-acting insulin intravenously or intramuscularly. (The insulin dose is determined by the size of the patient: big person, bigger dose; the height of the blood glucose: under 25 mmol/l lower dose, over 25 mmol/l higher dose; and the presence of infection: infected give a bigger dose.) Make sure that your note for the admitting officer contains details of the blood glucose, the insulin dose, and the time it was given.

Evidence of infection anywhere is also a danger sign. Infections in people with diabetes require prompt treatment which usually needs to be more intensive and longer lasting than in those without diabetes. As metabolic chaos can rapidly ensue during an infection, any patient with more than a minor infection should be assessed in hospital. ALL patients with ANY evidence of foot infection should be assessed by the diabetes team same day. Remember that the blood glucose rises rapidly in the presence of infection. A patient's insulin dose may double and people usually controlled on oral hypoglycaemic drugs may need insulin.

Pregnant women should be managed by a specialist diabetes team. Any problems with diabetes management should be referred on the same day to the diabetes team.

It may be difficult to assess elderly patients clinically; they may have severe hyperglycaemia with little clinical evidence. Have a low threshold for seeking hospital assessment of a hyperglycaemic elderly person. The same applies to young children.

Diabetes can make the treatment of any other illness more difficult and most other illnesses can cause hyperglycaemia. The presence of diabetes may determine the outcome of a co-existing illness. Such patients who become hyperglycaemic should be assessed in hospital. It is often better to refer the patient via the diabetes team who can then co-ordinate care with other disciplines. Alternatively, notify the diabetes team when referring a patient so that they can help to supervise the diabetes care.

Does the patient have symptoms of hyperglycaemia?

The symptoms of hyperglycaemia are mainly thirst, polyuria, and nocturia. The patient may also have general malaise and lethargy. These symptoms are unpleasant and the hyperglycaemia needs treating quickly. The blood glucose level at which they occur varies from person to person and some people appear to adapt to persistently high blood glucose concentrations. If the patient's only problem is symptomatic hyperglycaemia and they are not ill in other ways, they can usually be managed at home by the GP and/or the diabetes team. Treatment needs to be started or adjusted on the day the patient is seen, and the patient should be reviewed within a week. They should be give a contact number for immediate help if their condition deteriorates. If there is no response despite further treatment adjustment help should be sought from the diabetes team.

Management of diabetic ketoacidosis

This is still a major cause of death in people with insulin-treated diabetes under the age of 50 years. It is a preventable condition. Ketoacidosis must be treated promptly and effectively. It should always be managed in hospital.

Symptoms of diabetic ketoacidosis are vomiting, epigastric pain, thirst, polyuria, weakness, lethargy or malaise, and weight loss. Patients rarely complain of altered respiration. The most prominent symptom is vomiting—a feature which always signals danger in diabetes.

Signs of diabetic ketoacidosis may be few. Young people often tolerate it well. There may be a smell of ketones (rotten apples), a warm, dry skin, dehydration, tachycardia, and hyperventilation. Hypotension (postural or lying), poor peripheral circulation with cold peripheries, and alteration of conscious level or coma, are signs of severe fluid depletion and poor prognosis. There may also be the signs of a precipitating event such as infection.

Ketoacidotic patients should be transferred to hospital immediately by emergency ambulance. If the blood glucose is over 15 mmol/l give 4–10 units of clear, short-acting insulin intravenously or intramuscularly as described on p. 110 while awaiting transfer. If available, infuse normal (150 mmol/l, 0.9%) saline, 500 ml per hour, intravenously during transfer.

Management of hyperglycaemia

This section assumes that other urgent treatment has been initiated and that other problems (see Table 11.1) have been addressed. It is difficult to write because management which seems appropriate in theory is not always practical.

Insulin-treated patients

Every person with diabetes has one-off highs. These can be ignored. If the blood glucose is over 11 mmol/l for three or more days and any underlying condition (e.g. premenstrual state) has not resolved, action should be taken.

Check the blood glucose measuring technique. Check that you and the patient are both talking about the same insulin and the same doses. Observe insulin drawing up (or pen use), injection sites, injection process (is it too shallow, does insulin leak out). If these are all satisfactory, consider whether it is appropriate to increase the insulin, decrease the food, or increase regular exercise—or all three.

Acute hyperglycaemia in ill people

Increase insulin This usually occurs in the context of illness, for example an infection. An example of sick day rules for a person with diabetes is shown in Table 11.3. Agree sick day rules for each patient on insulin before they need them.

Chronic hyperglycaemia in 'well' people

Increase insulin Consider the time of peak action and length of action of the insulin acting at the time of hyperglycaemia. Increase one type of insulin at one injection time, wait 2 days for short-acting insulin, 3 days for intermediate-acting insulin, and 5 days for long-acting insulin, and review. Make further changes as appropriate. It is usual to increase the insulin by two units at a time (one unit in patients on less than 20 units a day). See Table 11.2.

Reduce carbohydrate food

The amount eaten at main meals may be reduced, or the food may be redistributed. It is unwise to stop snacks, and the pre-bedtime snack should never be stopped. People who have to get home from work (especially if driving or cycling) should always have a mid-afternoon snack. See Table 11.4.

Increase exercise

It is regular exercise within the training zone (see p. 116) which will help to reduce the blood glucose long term. Many people feel unable to make this commitment but it can be explored. Making an effort to walk regularly and use the stairs help will.

Patients on oral hypoglycaemic drugs

If the patient is hyperglycaemic on maximal doses of oral agents then they need insulin and this should be started without delay (see p. 77).

Increase oral hypoglycaemics

Unlike insulin in which there is no upper limit, oral hypoglycaemics have a maximum range. There is no benefit and possible harm in exceeding this. The dose should be increased gradually and with care not to induce hypoglycaemia at other times. It is often better to look at the food pattern if there is isolated hyperglycaemia during the day. All hypoglycaemic drugs may be effective when given once daily. Chlorpropamide should always be given once daily, but as their dose increases the other agents should be given twice or thrice daily (at meal times).

Reduce carbohydrate food

The required diet changes are similar to those for insulin-treated patients, although people on oral hypoglycaemic drugs need snacks less commonly. For people on oral

---

Table 11.2 Insulin increase

Time of high blood glucose	Insulin dose to increase
Before breakfast	Pre-dinner or pre-bed intermediate/long*-acting
Before lunch	Pre-breakfast short-acting
Before main evening meal (dinner)	Pre-breakfast intermediate/long*-acting Pre-lunch short-acting
Before bed	Pre-dinner short-acting Pre-breakfast long*-acting

* This assumes the patient is injecting a longer-acting insulin (Ultratard, for example) once a day.

Table 11.3 Sick day rules for a person with insulin-treated diabetes
If you are ill your blood glucose will usually rise as your body releases emergency hormones. This means that you will probably need more insulin than usual, even if you are not eating.

1. Measure your blood glucose 6-hourly; that is, before each meal time and before bed. Test your urine for ketones.

2. DO NOT STOP YOUR USUAL INSULIN
   Be prepared to inject extra insulin after each blood test.

Blood glucose	Clear, short-acting insulin (adapt the dose to the patient)
Below 11 mmol/l	No extra units
11.1–15 mmol/l	4 extra units
Over 15 mmol/l	6 extra units

3. If you cannot eat, drink plenty of fluid. Try to keep your carbohydrate intake up by drinking milk with added sugar, Lucozade, Coca Cola, Pepsi Cola, or other sugary drinks, unless your blood glucose is over 15 mmol/l.

4. CALL FOR HELP SOONER RATHER THAN LATER
   If your blood glucose is over 25 mmol/l on two occasions.
   If your blood glucose is over 11 and your urine shows ketones.
   If you are vomiting and unable to keep fluids down.
   If you feel too ill to measure your blood glucose.
   If you do not know what to do.

YOUR HELP TELEPHONE NUMBER IS:

This table may be photocopied for use by patients only. © Dr Rowan Hillson. From *Practical diabetes care*, Oxford University Press, 2002.

Table 11.4 Carbohydrate reduction to lower blood glucose

Time of high glucose level	Carbohydrate food to reduce
Mid-morning	Breakfast
Before lunch	Mid-morning snack/breakfast
Mid-afternoon	Lunch
Before main evening meal	Mid-afternoon snack/lunch
Before bed	Main evening meal

hypoglycaemics who are overweight, reduction in diet is the best way of improving glycaemic balance. See Table 11.4.

Increase exercise

Exercise should be regular and take place under the conditions described in Chapter 12. Elderly patients should be particularly careful to start an exercise programme gradually.

Summary

- Hyperglycaemia means blood glucose concentrations above the target zone (normally 4–8 mmol/l) for the each patient.
- In an acute situation, the level of the blood glucose is less important than the patient's condition.
- Ill patients should be transferred to hospital regardless of their blood glucose. Hyperglycaemia in pregnant women, elderly patients, and children should be managed in hospital.
- Patients with severe symptoms need prompt treatment.
- Diabetic ketoacidosis is a medical emergency requiring urgent treatment in hospital. It is preventable.
- Causes of hyperglycaemia are insufficient insulin or hypoglycaemic pills, excess food, too little exercise, infection, injury—accidental or surgical, myocardial infarction, menstruation, pregnancy, emotional stress, and drugs.
- Treatment of hyperglycaemia includes treating the cause if possible, and controlling the glucose by increasing hypoglycaemic therapy, reducing food, or increasing exercise.
- If the glucose cannot be controlled, seek the diabetes team's help early.

Chapter 12

Exercise

Exercise is good for people with diabetes. Regular exercise may, indeed, prevent or delay the onset of non-insulin-dependent diabetes. Regular exercise improves blood glucose balance in non-insulin-dependent diabetes and can do so in insulin-dependent diabetes if appropriate insulin dosage adjustments are made. Exercise increases insulin sensitivity, improves glucose tolerance, and in conjunction with a diet, helps weight reduction. Regular exercise also reduces the risk of coronary heart disease. It makes many people feel good.

In order to derive full benefit from exercise it should be regular—at least 20–30 minutes most days. The aim should be to keep the heart rate within the training zone (Table 12.1). This is between 60 and 85 per cent of the maximum heart rate. The heart rate should not exceed the maximum, calculated by subtracting the age from 220.

Exercise does not have to be weight lifting or marathon running. A brisk walk will maintain the pulse rate within the training zone. Furthermore, exercise which does not reach the training zone such as gardening or gentle swimming can be helpful in improving well-being and maintaining a full range of joint movement.

Exercise, insulin, and glucose

In a non-diabetic, exercising muscles first use their stored glycogen. Glucose is then taken up from the bloodstream as required for continued exercise. As the blood glucose concentration falls, pancreatic insulin release is reduced and glucose is released from the liver glycogen stores to 'top up' the blood glucose concentration. If carbohydrate has been eaten, this will be absorbed into the bloodstream and insulin will be released if necessary to store it in the liver and/or facilitate its use by the exercising muscles. Liver glycogenolysis will cease while the glucose derived from the meal is distributed. However, if exercise continues and the blood glucose level falls, insulin release will fall and liver glycogenolysis will again release glucose into the circulation.

This process can still occur in a person with diabetes treated by diet alone, and, to a large extent in metformin-treated patients. However, as soon as sulphonylureas or particularly insulin injections are introduced, the fine tuning of glucose balance in exercise is disturbed.

In a person with insulin-treated diabetes who exercises, the effects on blood glucose and other biochemistry, such as lipids, depend on the amount of circulating insulin and how much food has been eaten. The crucial difference between the diabetic and non-diabetic athlete is that there is no fine on/off control of insulin release.

Table 12.1 The training zone

Age (years)	Training zone—heart rate (beats/minute)		
	60%	85%	Maximum
15	123	174	205
20	120	170	200
25	117	166	195
30	114	162	190
35	111	157	185
40	108	153	180
45	105	149	175
50	102	145	170
55	99	140	165
60	96	136	160
65	93	132	155
70	84	119	140
75	87	123	145
80	84	119	140

To derive greatest benefit from exercise the heart rate should be within the training zone for 20 minutes or longer, most days. At first aim for the lower end of the training zone—60 per cent, or lower in someone who has not exercised recently. Do not use for people with autonomic neuropathy.

Someone who is insulin-deficient is likely to have a high blood glucose. Exercise will further increase the blood glucose as the stress hormone response releases glucose from the liver. As the exercise continues the muscles take up glucose from the bloodstream. However, this effect is unlikely to outweigh that of hepatic glucose release. Lipolysis, which occurs in prolonged exercise to provide free fatty acids as an additional fuel, may be followed by ketone formation in insulin deficiency. Any food eaten will merely serve to exacerbate the hyperglycaemia. Thus exercise may worsen hyperglycaemia and promote ketosis in an insulin-deficient person.

In someone who has a large subcutaneous reservoir of injected insulin, hypoglycaemia may ensue. As before, the exercising muscles will use their stored glycogen. The presence of insulin ensures good glucose uptake by the exercising muscles. However, high plasma insulin concentrations inhibit glucose release from the liver thereby further reducing the blood glucose concentration. Hypoglycaemia rapidly ensues. This situation can be prevented by eating carbohydrate which will be absorbed and top up the blood glucose level as exercise proceeds.

In patients taking sulphonylureas, the drugs enhance pancreatic insulin release, as well as improving tissue glucose uptake. They may thus produce hyperinsulinaemia and can cause exercise-induced hypoglycaemia.

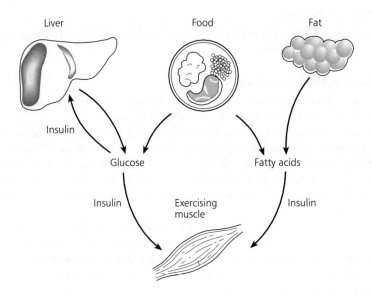

	At rest	**Brief exercise**	**Longer exercise**
Food	Glucose and fat absorbed into the blood	Glucose and fat absorbed into the blood	Less glucose and fat absorbed as some blood diverted to muscle
Insulin normal	Released from the pancreas according to blood glucose	Less insulin released from pancreas as glucose falls	
diabetic	Released from the injection site	More released from injection site as circulation to muscles and skin increases	
Liver	Stores glucose as glycogen*	Starts to release glucose ^	Releases a lot of glucose ^
Fat	Stores fatty acids*	Starts to release fatty acids ^	Releases a lot of fatty acids ^
Muscle	Stores glucose as glycogen*	Converts glycogen to glucose for energy ^	Takes up glucose and fatty acids and uses them for energy*

* Needs insulin
^ Blocked by insulin

Fig. 12.1 Exercise, food, and insulin

Helping people with diabetes to exercise safely

Controlling the blood glucose

Diet-treated diabetes

No special measures need to be taken regarding blood glucose balance if the glucose is well-controlled on diet alone.

Oral hypoglycaemic treatment

Metformin alone usually presents no problem, although if insulin sensitivity increases and weight is lost, a smaller dose of metformin may be needed.

Unexpected or vigorous exercise in patients taking sulphonylureas occasionally causes hypoglycaemia which may be prolonged. In this case, the person should check his blood glucose during or after exertion and eat some carbohydrate if necessary. If hypoglycaemia ensues the person should eat a series of small snacks until he is sure that the blood glucose has stabilized. The blood glucose must be checked regularly for at least 24 hours.

If the exercise is planned, it is better to reduce the dose of sulphonylurea before the exertion so that hypoglycaemia may be prevented. If too much carbohydrate is eaten to cover the exertion, excess insulin will be released and this may compound any late exercise-induced hypoglycaemia. If the exercise is regular, a long-term reduction in sulphonylurea dosage may be possible.

Insulin-treated diabetes

Exercise is a common cause of hypoglycaemia. For unexpected or vigorous exercise, refined carbohydrate snacks should be eaten before exercise and, if necessary, half-way through and afterwards. Blood glucose testing must be used to allow the person to assess what is happening as the symptoms of hypoglycaemia can be concealed beneath the sweating, tachycardia, and breathlessness of exercise. It is theoretically helpful to eat some high-fibre carbohydrate as well, but this may 'lie heavily on the stomach' of the athlete and reduce performance.

For planned exercise, the insulin acting during the time of exertion should be reduced beforehand. If the extent of the exertion is unknown (as in learning a new sport) it is better to reduce the insulin by about 20 per cent for the first few occasions. The insulin should be injected away from any exercising muscle. At the mealtime pre-ceding the exercise more high-fibre carbohydrate should be eaten unless this makes the person uncomfortable while exercising, in which this case a glucose- or sucrose-containing drink or snack before, during, and after (e.g. mini-chocolate bars such as *Mars*) can top up the blood glucose level during and after exercise. There must be no risk of hypoglycaemia while swimming or driving home from the pool or sports field. The next meal should contain more high-fibre carbohydrate than usual to prevent sub-sequent hypoglycaemia. The next dose of insulin may also need to be reduced after vigorous or endurance exercise. Hypoglycaemia may occur up to 24 hours after exercise.

There is no simple calculation for the amount of insulin dose reduction and the amount of extra carbohydrate. Each person has to work it out for themselves. The key is finger-prick blood glucose estimation. This should be four times a day (before each meal and before bed) and also immediately before and after the exercise until it has become familiar. As people train regularly, they will need less extra food for exercise and less insulin reduction.

Glucose control in dangerous activities

This applies especially to people on insulin injections. There are some sports in which the individual could die if they become confused or comatose (e.g. subaqua diving, hang-gliding). Other sports involve taking responsibility for others, either as coach or leader, or in sharing safety (e.g. belaying a climber). There is little or no margin for error and the individual must be certain that hypoglycaemia will not occur.

The insulin dose which acts during the activity must be reduced (20 per cent for most people, 50 per cent if hypoglycaemia prone or no warning of hypoglycaemia). The last meal preceding the activity should contain more carbohydrate than usual. If there has been a long preparation time for the activity and especially if this in itself has involved exercise (e.g. rowing out to a diving point, walking to the base of a climbing route) an appropriate double snack should be eaten and before starting the hazardous activity the blood glucose must be checked. If it is below 6 mmol/l an additional snack must be eaten and the blood glucose should be rechecked after 15–30 minutes. Immediately before starting the activity (e.g. just before putting foot to rock, or jumping into the water) two to four glucose tablets should be eaten. The aim is for the activity to take place on a rising glucose—rising from gut absorption which is independent of insulin concentration.

The same principles can be applied for situations in which hypoglycaemia could let the person down (e.g. in a competition) or let others down (e.g. team games). The difficulty lies in balancing freedom from hypoglycaemia, safety, and impairment of performance because of hyperglycaemia. Each sportsman has to spend some time experimenting for themselves. The only rule is start sugary and then fine tune.

Looking after the body

Any person starting an exercise programme needs to consider whether they are fit enough for their chosen activity, or whether it is safe for them to work towards attaining an appropriate standard of fitness for that activity. Also, remember that people with diabetes are more likely to have coronary heart disease than the general population (women as well as men) and that they may have diabetic tissue damage which could be further damaged by exercise.

Any patient in whom cardiac disease is suspected should have this investigated, probably by a cardiologist, before starting an exercise programme. Exercise is good for people with coronary heart disease, but only if it is appropriately graded and after any treatment required has been instituted. The American Diabetes Association advises that an exercise ECG may be helpful before starting an exercise programme (see Table 12.2). (It should be noted that this may not identify all those at risk.) As diabetes may modify cardiac symptoms these cannot necessarily be used as a guide to the degree of exercise that can be undertaken.

Table 12.2 Recommendations for an exercise ECG before a vigorous exercise programme

- Anyone over 35 years old
- Type 2 diabetes of > 10 years' duration
- Type 1 diabetes of > 15 years' duration
- Presence of any additional risk factor for coronary artery disease
- Presence of microvascular disease including microalbuminuria
- Peripheral vascular disease
- Autonomic neuropathy

Note A normal exercise ECG does not completely exclude coronary artery disease

Based on American Diabetes Association (1998) *Diabetes Care*, 21 (Suppl. 1), S40–4.

The diabetic foot is always vulnerable. In addition to standard foot care advice (see p. 149), those planning anything which involves walking or running or foot use should discuss appropriate foot wear (shoes and socks) with their chiropodist. Rubs and blisters are common in sport and neuropaths need to take especial care to avoid these while exercising. Running or jogging may exacerbate pressure areas and increase callus formation. Patients with Charcot change should exercise only under the guidance of their orthopaedic surgeon—just running on the spot can cause multiple fractures. Patients with peripheral vascular disease should keep their feet warm in cold weather—frost-bite can occur in Britain. Athletes' foot should be sought and treated. Foot hygiene must be scrupulous.

Proliferative retinopathy is a contraindication to exercise and to any activity involving lifting or staining. Until the ophthalmologist has confirmed that new vessels have regressed after treatment, any exertion could cause blindness from vitreous haemorrhage.

Questions for would-be exercisers and their tutors

These guidelines were originally drawn up by the author and subsequently modified with the help of members of the Diabetes UK (formerly BDA) Sports Working Party.

The person with diabetes

Can I do this activity? How fit am I?

You should always discuss exercise with your doctor.

- Is your exercise tolerance good? (Can you walk upstairs easily, run for a bus, mow the lawn for example?)

- Has your doctor told you to avoid any activities?

- Do you have diabetic eye disease, foot problems, heart disease, or other diabetic tissue damage? If yes, discuss exercise with your doctor.

- Following a heart attack you should avoid vigorous exercise for two months limiting your exercise to walking unless otherwise advised by your doctor.

♦ People with active new vessel disease of the eye should avoid excessive exertion until the eyes have been adequately treated. If you exercise too strenuously it can precipitate a bleed from these new vessels into the eye.

♦ If you have foot ulcers you should avoid weight bearing altogether on the affected foot. If you have a poor nerve supply or poor blood supply to your feet you should have your feet checked regularly by a state registered chiropodist.

Is my blood glucose balance under control?

♦ Do you know how to adjust your diet and treatment for different exercise levels? If not, ask your diabetes adviser.

♦ Do you take insulin or pills which may cause hypoglycaemia? If so, can you recognize and treat hypoglycaemia?

♦ Do you have hypoglycaemia often or without warning? If yes, consult your diabetes adviser.

Can I do this particular exercise safely?

♦ Does it involve short bursts of activity or prolonged, endurance exertion?

♦ Can you eat, take your treatment (if necessary), and test your blood glucose during the exercise?

♦ Can you keep food and diabetes equipment with you? Have you planned what to do if you become hypoglycaemic?

♦ How easy would it be for you to predict your energy expenditure and plan your eating and treatment before, during, and after exercise?

♦ If the activity is done outdoors what would happen if you needed assistance? Are you alone or with others? Are you close to a telephone or transport?

♦ Does it involve heat or cold, heights or depths, water or air? All of these can influence your blood glucose balance in addition to the exercise.

Is this sport or activity suitable for me?

There are regulations for some sports which relate to people with diabetes. Diabetes UK has a list of most of them. Ask your doctor whether he/she think this sport is appropriate for you.

The person supervising the activity

Can a person with diabetes do it safely?

♦ Do you understand what diabetes is and what it means? Are you aware of the different types of diabetes and their treatment?

♦ Are there regulations about people with diabetes doing this activity—do they apply here?

♦ The main risks are hypoglycaemia and the effects of tissue damage. Do you understand what hypoglycaemia is and how to recognize it? Hypoglycaemia, which sometimes causes confusion or coma, may not only affect the individual, but others involved in the activity, by-standers, and those involved in rescue.

- If the person becomes hypoglycaemic will he be a danger to himself or others? If yes, will you and he be able to recognize the warning symptoms, and will he be able to eat and cure the hypoglycaemia? If he does become seriously hypoglycaemic can you safeguard him (and others) and treat/rescue him if required?

Can this person with diabetes do it safely?

- Is he physically and mentally fit enough to start this activity?
- Have you gone through pp. 120–1 with the person?
- Can he adjust his diabetic treatment and diet to enjoy this activity safely without losing control of his diabetes?

Can I supervise him?

- Do I, personally, feel competent to supervise him this activity? Will I need additional help?

Summary

- Exercise is good for people with diabetes.
- Patients on sulphonylureas or insulin should reduce their medication and may often need to eat extra carbohydrate to fuel exercise.
- Take care to avoid hypoglycaemia, especially in high-risk sports.
- Consult Diabetes UK for further advice about individual sports.

Chapter 13

Diabetic tissue damage

In most people's minds diabetes is sugar trouble. Yet most of the problems of diabetes arise, not from the ups and downs of the glucose concentration but from its many tissue complications. Diabetes is a chronic multisystem disorder of which one manifestation is hyperglycaemia.

The tissue complications of diabetes are preventable and while we still have much to learn about the causes of diabetic tissue damage, we can at least work on reducing the damage due to factors we have identified. Diabetes is for life. The quality of that life and its extent will be largely determined by the development of tissue damage and its extent. Only half the people with Type 1 diabetes diagnosed before the age of 30 survive beyond the age of 50 years. The mortality rate for Type 1 diabetes is about five times that of their peers. For people with Type 2 diabetes the situation is unclear. They are probably about twice as likely to die early as their peers. However, the mortality and morbidity of diabetes is improving with modern care.

Diabetic tissue damage is usually divided into that which occurs only (or predominantly) in diabetes and that which is commoner in people with diabetes but does occur in others.

Microvascular disease—thickening of the basement membrane of capillaries causing leakage or blockage to the transfer of nutrients and waste substances, is virtually specific to diabetes. This is associated with retinopathy, nephropathy, and neuropathy. These and other changes, such as cheiroarthropathy and dermopathy, may be linked to glycosylation of proteins (see p. 62).

Macrovascular disease—atherosclerosis—is common in Western man, but is more frequent in people with diabetes.

Table 13.1 Tissue complications of diabetes

Eye—retinopathy, maculopathy, cataract, squint
Ear—deafness
Kidneys—nephropathy, renal failure, chronic pyelonephritis
Nerves—peripheral neuropathy, autonomic neuropathy, mononeuropathy, proximal motor neuropathy
Heart—ischaemic heart disease, cardiac failure
Legs—peripheral vascular disease
Brain—stroke, transient ischaemic attacks
Feet—ulcer, infection, gangrene, amputation
Skin—dermopathy, necrobiosis lipoidica
Ligaments—Dupuytren's contracture, cheiroarthropathy
Skeletal system—Charcot joint.

Table 13.2 Prevention of diabetic tissue damage

Treatment must be safe and practical for each patient

Help people with diabetes to learn how to work with the diabetes team:

- to reduce the risk of developing diabetic tissue damage
- to recognize tissue damage early, if present
- to slow deterioration of existing tissue damage

Reduce risk factors

- Stop smoking
- Keep the blood pressure below 130/80
- Keep the HbA1$_c$ between 4.5 and 6.4%*
- Keep the cholesterol below 5 mmol/l
- Keep the triglyceride below 2.3 mmol/l
- Treat microalbuminuria
- Keep the body mass index between 18 and 25 kg/m^2
- Exercise regularly
- Avoid added salt

* Or your laboratory's normal range

As most medical and nursing training relates to body systems the following discussion of tissue damage is considered by system rather than aetiology. In most instances symptoms are a late feature of diabetic complications. By the time the patient is aware of a problem it may be too late to treat it. Therefore a major part of diabetes care is screening patients for evidence of tissue damage and for risk factors of tissue damage (Table 13.2).

The eye

If you are planning to perform eye screening on your diabetic patients you must be confident in the use of the ophthalmoscope and know how to interpret what you see. Essential reading is *Diabetic eye disease* by Kritzinger and Taylor (1984) from which some of the following information has been taken with permission. Most diabetic eye clinics are happy to provide practical experience and teaching. Vision is so precious that the only safe rule must be, if in doubt, refer.

Diabetic eye disease is common. After 20 years of diabetes virtually every Type 1 patient, and most with Type 2 diabetes will have retinopathy. Before this, the incidence depends largely on the age of onset of diabetes and the type of diabetes. Type 1 patients diagnosed under the age of 30 years are unlikely to have retinopathy on diagnosis but develop it steadily after about three years. About one in five patients with maturity-onset Type 2 diabetes will have retinopathy at diagnosis.

Table 13.3 Eye problems in diabetes

Orbits	Fungal infections via sinus (rare)
Lids	Ptosis, inflammation
Eye muscles*	Mononeuropathy causing squint
Cornea	Reduced sensitivity, scratches, ulcers
Iris	Rubeosis iridis, **neovascular glaucoma**
Lens	**Cataract**, refraction problems
Vitreous	Posterior detachment
Retina	**Diabetic retinopathy**, lipaemia retinalis, central retinal vein occlusion
Optic nerve*	Swelling (papilloedema), optic atrophy

Conditions in **bold** are most likely to threaten vision
* Exclude other causes before attributing to diabetes
Adapted from Cavallerano (1990) and Ariffin *et al.* (1992)

Diabetic eye disease is the commonest cause of blindness among people of working age in the Western world.

Preventing diabetic eye disease

Factors which have been implicated are high blood glucose, hypertension, smoking, the contraceptive pill, and alcohol. Of these, high blood glucose and hypertension have definite links, the others are less clear. Diabetic retinopathy may progress rapidly during pregnancy.

Hyperglycaemia

Patients with persistent hyperglycaemia are much more likely to develop diabetic retinopathy than those with near-normal blood glucose levels. Normalization of the blood glucose slows the rate of development of retinopathy. However, it seems sensible to reduce the blood glucose gradually, over 4–8 weeks say, as a sudden return to normal may worsen retinopathy in the short-term.

Hypertension

This can cause a retinopathy in its own right, but uncontrolled hypertension may be associated with severe diabetic retinopathy. It has been suggested that lisinopril may reduce retinopathy.

Other factors

Pregnant women must have their eyes screened as soon as pregnancy is diagnosed and again later in pregnancy. It is probably sensible to avoid oral contraceptives in women with marked background or proliferative retinopathy. Smoking should be stopped anyway, and excess alcohol intake is inadvisable.

Screening—eyes

◆ Every patient with diabetes should attend their free annual eye check with an ophthalmic optician or optometrist. This is in addition to screening for diabetic eye disease by a doctor, optometrist, or nurse specifically trained in diabetic eye examination.

Try to alternate appointments so that someone checks the patient's eyes every 6 months.

◆ Screen all patients on diagnosis of diabetes and annually thereafter.

◆ Check every patient's visual acuity with a Snellen chart. Use pin-hole correction if acuity is worse than 6/6 in either eye.

◆ Examine every patient's lens and retina through dilated pupils (tropicamide 0.5 per cent or 1 per cent) using an ophthalmoscope. Do not dilate the pupils if the person has glaucoma, a family history of glaucoma, or has had eye surgery. Alternatively, ensure all patients have a retinal photograph in an ophthalmologist-approved retinal screening system.

If you cannot dilate the pupils, or if the visual acuity is worse than 6/9 despite pin-hole correction, refer the patient to an ophthalmologist. (NB If the patient is hyper-glycaemic, it is advisable to retest the eyes after the blood glucose has returned to normal—hyperglycaemia may cause temporarily blurred vision.) If the pin-hole resolves the impairment of visual acuity advise the patient to visit an ophthalmic optician or optometrist. Patients should not buy new spectacles until their blood glucose level is stable, preferably near normal.

Warning symptoms

◆ Deterioration in vision—examine the eyes immediately as described above.

◆ 'Floaters', blobs or wisps across the vision. The patient may have had a vitreous haemorrhage (Fig. 13.1). Examine the eye as described under 'Screening' but if you cannot see anything abnormal refer to an ophthalmologist for urgent assessment. Otherwise follow the procedure below.

Squint

This may occur acutely, often with associated pain, as a sign of diabetic mononeuro-pathy. The 3rd, 4th, or 6th nerve may be affected. In 3rd nerve palsy due to diabetes, pupillary function is often intact. The squint may gradually resolve. Beware the coincidental brain tumour. Refer patients with a new squint to the medical on-call team or a neurologist same day.

Lens

If the patient has a cataract in either eye and they have impaired visual acuity or you cannot see the retina, refer them to an ophthalmologist. Patients under 30 with cataracts should be seen by an ophthalmologist that week; acutely developing juvenile cataract can cause blindness within days.

The macula

To see this ask the patient to look at your light (a macular beam is kindest if your ophthalmoscope has one). This is the area of best vision so problems here require urgent treatment.

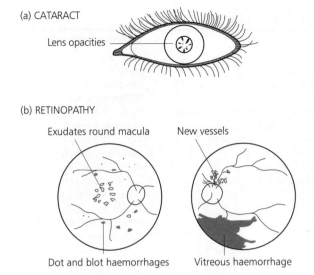

Fig. 13.1 Diabetic eye problems: (a) cataract, (b) retinopathy

Macular oedema If the little pink dot which marks the fovea is blurred or if the whole macula appears swollen, the patient should be seen by an ophthalmologist within a month. Because the patient's problem is at the fovea, using a pin-hole to correct visual acuity may make it worse.

Macular exudates If there is a ring of hard, yellow exudates around or near the macula this may impair the best vision. The patient should be seen by an ophthalmologist within a month.

The retina

Microaneurysms and blot haemorrhages These red dots and blots indicate background retinopathy (Fig. 13.1). This will not impede vision but may progress. If visual acuity is impaired despite pin-hole correction refer to an ophthalmologist. Otherwise, keep it under review every three to six months.

Hard exudates These are shiny, clearly defined, yellowish fatty exudates. It may be difficult to assess the degree of severity. Refer the patient to an ophthalmologist. An urgent referral is needed if these exudates are at the macula (see above).

Dilated veins A sign of diabetic ophthalmopathy. If the veins also have bulges and extra loops on them this means pre-proliferative retinopathy: such patients should see an ophthalmologist within a month.

Soft exudates These are like blobs of cotton wool—pale and poorly defined. Like veins with blobs and extra loops with which they are often seen, soft exudates are usually a sign of pre-proliferative retinopathy and such patients should see an ophthalmologist within a month.

Table 13.4 Eyes-urgent action

Problem	Ophthalmologist review
Sudden loss of vision	Same day
Retinal detachment	Same day
Central retinal vein occlusion	Same day
New vessels	Within one week
Haemorrhage inside eye (vitreous/pre-retinal)	Within one week
Rubeosis iridis (new vessels on iris)	Within one week
Cataract in patients under 30 years old	Within one week
Macular oedema	Within one month
Unexplained fall in visual acuity	Within one month
Hard exudates near fovea	Within one month
Severe retinopathy	Within one month
Dilated/tortuous veins	Within one month
Soft exudates	Within one month
Unexplained findings	Within one month
New squint or eye movement problems	Refer to Medical on-call team or neurologist same day

Sources of information include Affrin *et al.* (1992), (Kritzinger (1984), NICE Clinical Guideline E (2002), and Royal College of General Practitioners (2002).

New vessels These fine tangles of tiny vessels are most often seen near the optic disc but can occur anywhere including at the periphery of an otherwise normal looking fundus. Disc vessels are particularly likely to bleed. Neovascularization indicates proliferative retinopathy. Contact the ophthalmologist—the patient should be seen within a week.

Vitreous haemorrhage (Fig. 13.1) Vitreous haemorrhage should not happen—it is largely preventable. Bleeding occurs when the fragile new vessels are damaged. Red or black blobs ('tadpoles', 'floaters') or wisps float across the patient's vision. A big bleed may be like a curtain. The haemorrhage may clear, but some people may develop severe permanent visual impairment. Telephone the ophthalmologist for a same-day appointment. The more bleeding, the harder it may be to visualize the bleeding vessels and attempt to photocoagulate them.

Advanced eye disease Even if the interior of the eye appears completely disorganized with fibrous bands pulling on the retina and detaching it, vitreous surgery, and other specialist techniques may be helpful. Rubeosis may occur, that is new vessels on the iris causing glaucoma, but it may be treatable. Such patients should be seen by an ophthalmologist within a week.

Other retinal problems Thrombosis of retinal arteries and veins, and glaucoma are commoner in people with diabetes than the general population. They all require prompt ophthalmological advice.

Laser photocoagulation

The aim is to induce regression of new vessels and sometimes to seal leaking new vessels. It is also used to treat maculopathy. Laser treatment prevents severe visual impairment in the majority of patients although the results for maculopathy are less predictable because treatment is close to the macula. Patients should understand that laser treatment may not improve vision but it should stop major deterioration. The treatment is usually given in one or more 30–60 minute sessions as an out-patient. Local anaesthetic and dilating eye drops are used and the patient just has to remain still and concentrate while the treatment is given. Afterwards there is blurring of vision, photophobia, and sometimes eye discomfort or headache. Patients who complain of severe pain should be referred to the eye casualty service.

The ears

It is not always realized that hearing loss in diabetes may be due to 8th nerve neuropathy or microvascular disease. There is little information about this, but patients with hearing loss should always have a formal auditory assessment. It seems sensible to ensure that blood glucose balance is good as this is implicated in other microvascular disease.

The kidneys

After 15 years of diabetes about one in three people with Type 1 diabetes will have evidence of diabetic nephropathy. Fewer people with Type 2 diabetes are affected— estimates vary. Renal failure is the cause of death in 10 to 20 per cent of people with Type 1 diabetes, but only 1 to 2 per cent of those with Type 2 diabetes.

Preventing or slowing renal impairment

Hyperglycaemia

Persistent hyperglycaemia is linked with increased likelihood of developing nephropathy. Normalization of the blood glucose slows the rate of deterioration of renal function. This may be difficult to achieve without hypoglycaemia in patients with impaired renal function who should perform frequent finger-prick blood glucose testing. Most of these patients will end up on insulin although 50 per cent of people with diabetes who develop end-stage renal failure have Type 2 diabetes.

Hypertension

Tight control of hypertension slows deterioration of renal function in nephropaths. This means treating people whose blood pressure would not normally fall into the treatment range for non-diabetic people. In patients with known diabetic kidney disease the aim is to keep the blood pressure below 125/75 but be careful to avoid dizziness and falls in patients with severe postural hypotension due to autonomic neuropathy.

Treating microalbuminuria (see p. 54)

There is evidence that ACE inhibitors slow the progression of diabetic nephropathy if initiated when persistent microalbuminuria is detected. Test for microalbumin: creatinine ratio annually in patients without dipstick proteinuria. If the ratio is raised in two of three samples collected consecutively within one month, prescribe an ACE inhibitor e.g. Ramipril.

Low-salt diet

A reduction in sodium chloride intake may help control hypertension and reduce fluid retention.

Screening—kidneys

♦ Screen every patient at diagnosis of diabetes and annually thereafter.

♦ Screen by measuring urinary microalbumin concentrations (see p. 54).

♦ Screen by measuring plasma creatinine concentrations.

Warning symptoms or sings

♦ None: by the time symptoms and signs develop, severe renal impairment is present

♦ Hypoglycaemia or falling insulin or tablet dose

♦ Rising blood pressure

♦ Oedema.

Diabetic nephropathy

If the microalbumin concentration is raised check for infection (midstream urine microscopy and culture). If infection is present treat it and then repeat the micro-albumin estimation after the infection has settled. Cardiac failure may also produce microalbuminuria. If the creatinine is raised perform a creatinine clearance test. Note that small people or those with low muscle bulk should have creatinine levels at the lower end of the normal range. Do a creatinine clearance if their creatinine is in the upper half of the normal range.

It may take several years for microalbuminuria to progress to overt albuminuria and for other signs of renal impairment to develop. The rate of deterioration of renal function can be slowed down.

If the patient has albuminuria on Albustix, or reduced creatinine clearance, assess their kidneys further. Most of these patients will have diabetic nephropathy but it is important to distinguish those who do not. Examine the patient's fundi for retino-pathy—if this is absent it is unlikely that the patient has diabetic nephropathy. Is there a previous history of kidney disease, or a family history of renal problems? Do they have symptoms of recurrent urinary infection or prostatism, for example. Measure the blood pressure lying and standing. Check midstream urine microscopy and culture. If there is no infection measure the 24-hour urinary protein excretion. Request a renal ultrasound.

All patients with evidence of nephropathy should be seen by a diabetologist and a renal physician. Several centres now have joint renal diabetes clinics. Patients may need continuous ambulatory peritoneal dialysis (CAPD) or, less often, haemodialysis. CAPD has a 60 per cent three-year survival rate in diabetes. A quarter of patients entering some renal transplant programmes have diabetes. Transplants have over 60 per cent five-year survival.

Patients with diabetic nephropathy always have retinopathy and often have foot problems, neuropathy, vascular disease, and ischaemic heart disease. Many die from the latter rather than from their renal impairment.

Diabetic neuropathy

Diabetes can produce virtually any peripheral (sensory or motor) or autonomic neurological deficit. Because it is difficult to measure minor degrees of neuropathy, its frequency is difficult to establish. After 20 years of diabetes most people have evidence of impaired nerve function on detailed testing. About one in twelve people with newly diagnosed Type 2 diabetes have clinically detectable neuropathy.

Preventing or improving neuropathy

Hyperglycaemia

People with persistently high blood glucose levels are more likely to have peripheral neuropathy than those with normal glucose levels. Normalization of the glucose concentration (some authorities believe insulin should always be used) may relieve severe pain or abnormal feelings in neuropathy. Returning the glucose to normal slows worsening peripheral neuropathy and may also improve it but seems to have little effect on autonomic neuropathy.

Screening—nerves

♦ Screen every patient at diagnosis of diabetes and annually thereafter.

♦ Symptoms: numbness, tingling, weakness. There are often none

♦ Examination: muscle wasting
                    muscle weakness (if symptoms/wasting)

♦ Feet: light touch—cotton wool
          pressure—Monofilaments (10 g or less is normal)
          pin prick—Neurotips (Owen Mumford)
          vibration—tuning fork (C_0 pitch)
          position sense
          tendon reflexes—ankle, knee

♦ Blood pressure: lying and standing

Peripheral neuropathy

There are several nomenclatures which can be confusing. In practice they are not always clearly definable. From the patient's point of view it is important to know if any sensory modality is missing so as to be careful to avoid injury; if it hurts or feels peculiar; or if a muscle is weak or does not work.

The commonest form of neuropathy is loss or blunting of sensation in a 'sock' or sometimes 'glove' distribution. Different modalities may be differently affected.

Problems that arise are numbness so that rubbing or injury is not noticed, loss of temperature discrimination with a risk of burning, loss of position sense which, if severe, can make walking and balance difficult. Loss of vibration sense is an early sign of neuropathy but has no major clinical impact. This peripheral neuropathy may be accompanied by tingling or actual pain.

Single nerve lesions, with or without entrapment, are quite common. They include median and ulnar nerves and those serving eye movement (see p. 126).

Muscle weakness may be secondary to an individual nerve lesion (as above) or more diffuse. It can affect the thighs with marked wasting, weakness, and pain, or rarely be more extensive.

Many patients are unaware of the extent of their neuropathy until they are affected by one of its consequences such as a foot ulcer at the site of an unnoticed injury. A few are severely disabled by pain. Such patients should be referred to a diabetologist. The pain is sometimes relieved by minor analgesics, but if not, tricyclic antidepressants, carbamazepine, or phenytoin may help.

Obviously the most likely reason for neuropathy in someone with diabetes is diabetic tissue damage. However, it is important not to miss other treatable causes such as vitamin B_{12} deficiency, vitamin B_6 deficiency, alcohol excess, drugs, uraemia, collagen-vascular disease, and other conditions.

Warning for neuropathic patients

- Never walk barefoot
- Check shoes and socks for foreign bodies every time you put them on
- Never use a hot water bottle
- Check the bath-water temperature with a bath thermometer
- Always use an oven glove
- Inspect your feet every day.

Autonomic neuropathy

Two in five patients with diabetes have some evidence of autonomic neuropathy when tested in detail, but symptoms are uncommon. If the patient does have symptoms these may be unpleasant and the prognosis is poor. One in two patients with symptomatic autonomic neuropathy will be dead within 5 years. Symptoms include:

- postural hypotension
- altered sweating
- gastroparesis
- diarrhoea or constipation
- urinary retention
- impotence
- ankle swelling
- loss of hypoglycaemia warning
- sudden death

All patients with evidence of autonomic neuropathy should be referred to a consultant diabetologist.

Screening—autonomic neuropathy: symptomatic patients

Apart from blood pressure, tests for autonomic neuropathy are usually reserved for symptomatic patients. Some are complex. The following can be done with a sphygmomanometer and an ECG machine:

1 Lying and standing systolic blood pressure. Normal fall ≤ 10 mmHg; abnormal fall ≥ 30 mmHg.

2 Heart rate during and after Valsalva manoeuvre. Find pulse, ask patient to breathe in, then to try to push the breath out hard against a closed glottis for as long as they can. Count the pulse once they've started. Then count the rate as they relax afterwards. It is much easier with an ECG machine. Rate during/rate after: normal ≥ 1.21; abnormal ≤ 1.20. Do not do this in people with proliferative retinopathy.

3 Heart rate after standing '30:15 test'. Attach the ECG and make sure the patient will be able to get up easily. Once the ECG is recording continuously ask the patient to stand and mark the ECG as they start to do so. Calculate the ratio of the longest R—R interval (about the 30th beat after they start standing over the shortest R—R interval (about the 15th beat after they start standing): normal ≥ 1.04; abnormal ≤ 1.0.

These tests are fraught with practical difficulties (patients who find it hard to stand up, ECG leads fall off, etc.).

Postural hypotension

There may be a marked fall of blood pressure for some minutes after standing, with or without feelings of dizziness. Some patients have falls or blackouts. Some patients cannot even sit up in bed without fainting. Postural hypotension can be made worse by fluid depletion, hypotensive treatment, diuretics, nitrates and other vasodilators, psychotropic drugs (such as tricyclics).

Remove or reduce drugs worsening the situation and ensure adequate hydration. Compression stockings may help, as may fludrocortisone in severe cases.

Altered sweating

Patients may sweat less on the feet but more in the upper half of the body. This includes gustatory sweating—facial sweating precipitated by spicy or highly flavoured foods. Avoiding these foods may help. The lack of moisture in the feet may lead to dry skin and moisturizing cream can be used except between the toes.

Gastroparesis

Slow stomach emptying can cause abdominal discomfort, hypoglycaemia, and vomiting. In rare cases the vomiting may be debilitating and require hospital admission. Metoclopramide may improve stomach emptying. Oesophageal motility may also be abnormal and some patients may experience swallowing problems.

Diarrhoea or constipation

Either of these symptoms should be investigated in the usual way before attributing them to diabetic neuropathy. Diabetic diarrhoea can be distressing. It comes in bouts of days or weeks, with urgency, especially at night. Codeine or loperamide may help. In more severe cases a short trial of a broad spectrum antibiotic like neomycin is sometimes successful. The rationale is that this reduces bacterial overgrowth in the abnormal bowel. Constipation can be treated by continuing the high-fibre diet (but not if there is gastroparesis), plenty of soft fruit, and laxatives if needed.

Urinary retention

This occurs imperceptibly. The bladder slowly enlarges with an increasing post-miction volume. This forms a reservoir for infection. Once the patient is made aware of the problem, regular urination with pressure in the suprapubic region may help. If the person suffers recurrent urinary infections, prophylactic antibiotics such as trimethoprim may be required. Other causes of urinary retention, such as prostatism, must be excluded. They may coincide.

Sudden death

This may obviously happen at any time but people with autonomic neuropathy are at especial risk if they become hypoxic or during anaesthesia. The anaesthetist should always be made aware that the patient has autonomic neuropathy and anaesthesia should be performed only in a hospital with full resuscitation and medical support.

Diabetic skin and musculoskeletal problems

Skin

Infection Minor skin infection may be the first clue to diabetes and can remain a problem. It ranges from boils to the more serious carbuncle. Pustules on the legs and elsewhere may also be staphylococcal in origin. Cellulitis, often streptococcal or staphylococcal, can spread very fast. Paronychia, especially related to ingrowing toenails, is common. Fungal infections, usually candida, affect the perineum and produce intertrigo in the groins and elsewhere in obese patients.

Diabetic dermopathy Shin spots are flat reddish-brown marks in the pretibial region. They may follow trauma but can emerge spontaneously. They do not require treatment.

Necrobiosis lipoidica diabeticorum Is not common. It occurs in about 3 patients with diabetes per 1000 per year. The lesions are red plaques with a purple edge and a yellowish centre which gradually becomes atrophic. They usually occur on the pretibial area and may remit spontaneously. The lesions are rarely a problem but young women may be very distressed by the cosmetic defect. Treatment is not always satisfactory. Steroids can be used on non-atrophic lesions and some authorities advocate nicotinic acid orally. Skin grafting may be successful.

Itching May be associated with perineal candidiasis.

Ligaments

Skin thickening can occur in diabetes but connective tissue thickening is more obvious in ligaments. Diabetes is associated with Dupuytren's contracture, similar problems in the feet, carpal tunnel syndrome, and cheiroarthropathy. Cheiroarthropathy is a tightening of the tendons in the hand so that fingers can no longer be pressed flat against those of the other hand when opposed. Joint mobility may be generally limited. Frozen shoulder and trigger finger are more common in people with diabetes than in the population at large.

Bones

People with diabetes can develop marked osteopenia. Loss of bone density may be most evident in the first few years after diagnosis of Type 1 diabetes. It seems to be linked to poor blood glucose balance. Patients with Type 2 diabetes may also have reduced bone density. Fractures of the femur may be more common in older people with diabetes than in non-diabetic people. Severe neuropathy and trauma may cause bone destruction and Charcot joints. Osteoarthrosis also appears to be more common. Thirteen per cent of people with rheumatoid arthritis also have diabetes.

Cardiovascular disease

- ◆ heart
- ◆ peripheral vascular disease
- ◆ hypertension
- ◆ cerebrovascular disease

Cardiovascular disease is about two to three times as common in people with diabetes as in the general population. Premenopausal diabetic women are about as likely to have a myocardial infarct as diabetic men. Diabetic men are over two times, diabetic women over three times, as likely to die from cardiovascular causes as the general population. About 70 per cent of people with diabetes die from cardiovascular disease (mostly coronary artery disease).

Prevention and reduction of cardiovascular risk

People with diabetes should pay attention to the same risk factors as those without diabetes. It seems likely that all these risk factors have a more detrimental effect on people with diabetes. The main risk factors are smoking, hypertension, obesity, and hyperlipidaemia.

It used to be thought that glucose concentrations were not directly linked with large vessel disease. However, the DCCT (see p. 29) showed a reduction in plasma cholesterol concentrations in the intensively treated patients and a trend towards less cardiovascular disease in those with near normoglycaemia. In UKPDS (see p. 29) patients with intensive glucose control on metformin had a lower risk of fatal myocardial infarct than these on conventional glucose control. However, the sulphonylurea and insulin groups did not show a significant reduction in cardiovascular events with intensive glucose lowering.

Smoking

Diabetic smokers have a similarly increased risk of cardiovascular disease to non-diabetics. Overweight, hypertensive diabetic women who are taking oral contraceptives are at especially high risk of cardiovascular complications. Studies have also shown that smokers were more likely to have nephropathy and retinopathy than non-smokers.

Obesity

Obesity is common in people with Type 2 diabetes and can occur in insulin-treated patients, especially if they are eating to keep up with their insulin. To help patients lose weight safely reduce their glucose-lowering treatment as they start their reduced calorie diabetes diet. Patients must be aware of the risk of hypoglycaemia. Some patients on insulin or oral hypoglycaemic drugs may be able to stop them if they lose weight. Patients treated by diet alone may need medication if they gain weight. Beware of the weight loss of uncontrolled diabetes. Remember to measure the patient's height—it is often forgotten. (See p. 47.)

Hypertension

This is discussed on page 140.

Hyperlipidaemia

Glucose is not the only biochemical problem in diabetes. Both cholesterol and trigly-ceride may be raised in diabetes. In addition, lipoproteins are glycosylated and this process may be involved in atherogenesis. Hyperlipidaemia can be defined as:

Cholesterol   > 5.0 mmol/l
HDL cholesterol < 0.9 mmol/l
LDL cholesterol > 3.0
Triglyceride   > 2.3 mmol/l

These values relate to a fasting sample.

Triglyceride The main lipid abnormality in diabetes is hypertriglyceridaemia. Plasma triglyceride is elevated in about a third of patients with Type 2 diabetes. Patients with Type 1 diabetes who are insulin-deficient also have high triglycerides. A few patients have extremely high plasma triglyceride levels and their serum is milky with chylomicrons. These patients may have eruptive xanthomata, abdominal pain, and pancreatitis, with malaise, tingling, and impaired cerebral function.

Cholesterol Total cholesterol is more likely to be raised in Type 2 patients than Type 1. HDL cholesterol has the same inverse relationship to coronary heart disease and other conditions due to atheroma as in non-diabetic people. HDL cholesterol is more often reduced in women with Type 2 diabetes than in men. The abnormalities related to HDL cholesterol are more closely linked with triglyceride than to total cholesterol.

Seek and treat secondary causes of hyperlipidaemia

Factors affecting triglyceride levels are:

- glucose control
- alcohol
- obesity
- liver disease
- chronic renal failure
- nephrotic syndrome
- thiazides
- beta blockers
- myeloma

Factors affecting cholesterol levels are:

- hypothyroidism   - eating disorders
- cholestasis   - diuretics
- nephrotic syndrome

Management of hyperlipidaemia in diabetes

Diet This should be low-fat, high-complex carbohydrate, high-soluble fibre, low-sugar diet, with weight reduction if required. Continue the diet for at least six weeks with vigorous encouragement before considering drugs. Keep alcohol to 21 units per week for men and 14 units per week for women.

Exercise (see Chapter 12).

Control glucose Control blood glucose in all cases.

Reducing cholesterol and triglyceride (see Appendix A, p. 214).

Lipid-lowering drugs

Encourage all diabetic patients with hyperlipidaemia to eat less fat, achieve optimal weight for their height, exercise regularly and safely, stop smoking, and control their glucose to near normal levels. Treat secondary causes. However, even if you do all this many diabetic patients will still have a cholesterol over 5 mmol/l and/or triglycerides over 2.3 mmol/l. We await the detailed results of a large primary prevention study including thousands of diabetic patients (the Heart Protection Study). However, evidence from this and more general population studies and from secondary prevention strongly suggests that medication should be used to reduce lipids in diabetic patients not known to have cardiac or vascular disease in whom lifestyle measures have failed. Lipid lowering reduces cardiovascular events in secondary prevention studies in diabetic groups (see Chapter 3). These patients should be given lipid-lowering drugs immediately.

Statins and fibrates can cause liver dysfunction, and all lipid-lowering drugs can cause gastrointestinal side-effects. All may interact with warfarin. None should be given to women of child-bearing potential unless they are using reliable contraception, although cholestyramine has been used in severe hypercholesterolaemia in pregnancy. Statins and fibrates can cause myalgia and, rarely, rhabdomyolysis. Avoid lipid-lowering drugs in patients with liver or biliary disease and exercise caution in those with renal disease. Hyperlipidaemia in transplant patients should be managed by specialist centres, as should familial hypercholesterolaemia.

In general, check liver function before starting statins or fibrates and twice in the first year or until one year after the last dose increase. Stop the drug if a liver enzyme (ALT or AST) is greater than three times the upper limit of normal. If the patient develops muscle pain, stop the drug and check creatine phosphokinase. If this is not elevated the drug can be restarted. Read individual drug data sheets. If the lipids fail to fall on a maximum dose of one drug (and the patient is taking it) they may need combination therapy with statins and fibrates. This should be initiated with specialist help as there is a greater risk of rhabdomyolysis and other side-effects.

Statins

Atorvastatin, fluvastatin, pravastatin, and simvastatin. These drugs are now first-line treatment for raised cholesterol. Simvastatin and pravastatin in particular have both been used in large, lengthy studies which included people with diabetes (see Chapter 3). Statins can lower LDL cholesterol by up to 40 per cent with a slight increase in HDL and reduction in triglyceride. Atorvastatin is the most potent triglyceride-reducing statin. Simvastatin at a dose of 80 mg daily can also lower triglyceride. Pravastatin is less likely to interact with warfarin than other statins. These drugs work best if taken before bed.

Fibrates

Bezafibrate, ciprofibrate, fenofibrate, and gemfibrozil. These drugs reduce both cholesterol and triglyceride and should be used as first-line agents in patients whose triglyceride is over 5 mmol/l with or without elevated cholesterol. They may also be used in patients with raised cholesterol and a triglyceride over 2.3 mmol/l, or in those with isolated hypercholesterolaemia who cannot tolerate statins.

Bile-acid sequestrants

Cholestyramine or colestipol. Use these if patients cannot tolerate other agents, or in combination for severe hypercholesterolaemia. However, bile-acid sequestrants often cause gastrointestinal side-effects and are poorly tolerated. Use in patients with high cholesterol but avoid if triglycerides are raised. Start very cautiously with half a sachet before a meal and increase gradually. Other medication should be taken one hour before or four hours after the bile-acid sequestrant. This medication may cause reduction in absorption of fat-soluble vitamins.

Soluble fibre

Ispaghula husk (Fybozest) increases soluble fibre in the gut and can reduce cholesterol. It may cause gastrointestinal side-effects but can be used as a 'natural' lipid-lowering agent for patients who prefer this or who cannot tolerate other drugs. Ispaghula should be introduced gradually. It may slow glucose absorption and cause hypoglycaemia.

Screening—cardiovascular

There is less consensus about the timing and frequency of some screening for cardio-vascular disease and its risk factors in diabetes than there is for microvascular disease. What is suggested is a compromise. (See *National Service Frameworks for Coronary Heart Disease* (2000).)

Heart

People with diabetes are more likely to have coronary atheroma than the general population. They also have cardiac small vessel disease with basement membrane

On diagnosis of diabetes check:

- Symptoms of cardiovascular disease (e.g. angina, intermittent claudication)
- Smoking history
- Family history of heart disease
- Height and weight
- Blood pressure
- Pulse
- Heart size, sounds, and evidence of failure
- Peripheral pulses
- ECG if hypertensive or evidence of cardiac disease (some doctors would screen all those with Type 2 diabetes)
- Chest X-ray if smoker, hypertensive, evidence of respiratory or cardiac disease, tuberculosis-prone
- Cholesterol and triglyceride

Screen patients annually (or as stated) thereafter:

- Cardiovascular symptoms
- Smoking
- Family history—new events?
- Weight (assess in relation to height)
- Blood pressure
- Peripheral pulses
- Cardiac examination if symptoms, otherwise every 5 years
- ECG if symptoms and every 5 years routinely
- Cholesterol and triglyceride (2 monthly if elevated, every year if normal)

thickening as in the retina. This probably contributes to the higher frequency of cardiomyopathy in people with diabetes, with or without coronary artery disease.

Angina

Some patients will present with classic symptoms of angina pectoris. In others with autonomic neuropathy the symptoms may be different or less pronounced, and there is a greater likelihood of silent ischaemia. Have a higher index of suspicion that cardiac disease may be present in such patients. The only symptom of myocardial ischaemia may be undue exertional tiredness or breathlessness. In patients in whom ischaemia is suspected and who do not show an acute myocardial infarct on their ECG, an exercise ECG should be done. As these patients may be difficult to diagnose and treat, a cardiologist's advice should be sought early. If the exercise ECG is positive it should be followed by coronary angiography.

Myocardial infarction

Myocardial infarction can occur at a younger age than in non-diabetic people, and in premenopausal women.

> A 25-year-old woman with Type 1 diabetes since childhood was admitted in diabetic ketoacidosis. She complained of chest pain. A 12-lead ECG showed widespread ST elevation. Shortly after admission she had a cardiac arrest from which she could not be resuscitated. At post-mortem she had very extensive myocardial infarction.

Unexplained hyperglycaemia or ketoacidosis may indicate silent myocardial infarction. If there is any suspicion of acute myocardial infarction the patient should be given an aspirin and transferred immediately to an emergency department. Diabetic patients with myocardial infarction are twice as likely to die as non-diabetic people. Like non-diabetic people, those with diabetes benefit from thrombolysis but the admitting team must be warned if the patient has proliferative retinopathy as thrombolytics could precipitate a vitreous haemorrhage.

Cardiac failure

This is common in people with diabetes, with or without symptoms of myocardial ischaemia. It may be preceded by a reduction in left ventricular function which can be found in asymptomatic young people and children with diabetes. Cardiac failure can cause hyperglycaemia and rising insulin requirements. It is important to control the blood glucose level as this may improve cardiac function. Hypoglycaemia, with its dramatic circulatory and electrolyte shifts should be avoided in cardiac patients. Reduce dietary sodium chloride.

Treatment of cardiac disease

Strongly discourage smoking. Encourage weight loss and a low-fat diet. Control hypertension and hyperlipidaemia if present. Control hyperglycaemia. Use the most appropriate drugs within the caveats below. As cardiac disease is more severe and more likely to prove fatal in people with diabetes it should be managed with greater therapeutic 'aggression' than in non-diabetic people, with earlier intervention, including coronary artery bypass grafting if indicated.

Diabetes and drugs used in cardiac disease

Many cardiac drugs have practical or theoretical problems in some people with diabetes and should be chosen with great care. However, diabetic patients should not be deprived of their benefits. See below (p. 142).

Aspirin Should be given to all patients with known coronary disease unless contra-indicated.

Hypertension

There is much debate about why people with diabetes are about two times more likely to have hypertension than non-diabetic people. Hypertension is found in one in three people with diabetes—or more. As with other tissue damage hypertension is uncommon

Table 13.5 Tests in people with hypertension

Electrolytes
Urate
Creatinine (clearance if raised)
Cholesterol and triglyceride
Full blood count
Urine—microalbumin, microscopy, culture if indicated
ECG
Chest X-ray
Consider renal ultrasound
(Urinary catecholamines and free cortisol etc. if indicated)

in people with newly diagnosed Type 1 diabetes but is frequent in those with Type 2 diabetes at diagnosis. Rare causes of hypertension (e.g. Cushing's syndrome, phaeochromocytoma, acromegaly) will be found slightly more often in people with diabetes than in the general population. Non-diabetic renal causes should be considered.

Several, slightly different definitions of hypertension in people with diabetes have been put forward over the past two years. The British Hypertension Society (p. 221) advises two or three readings per visit in a seated relaxed patient, taken at monthly intervals over a four to six-month period before diagnosing hypertension. Phase V (disappearance of sound) should always be used to determine diastolic pressure. The aim in the general population is a blood pressure below 140/85. They advise an aim of below 140/80 in diabetic patients. However, the Joint British Societies (see p. 28) advised a lower reading of below 130/80 under optimal conditions in diabetic patients, and this would seem more likely to protect the patient from cardiovascular and renal disease. However, this more rigorous level is harder to achieve and carries greater risk of postural hypotension and side-effects of medication. A realistic and safe target needs to be set for each patient (see p. 26).

Treatment

Help the patient to lose weight. Reduce their salt intake and consider other non-pharmacological measures such as stress reduction and relaxation. However, most patients will still need medication. Angiotensin converting enzyme (ACE) inhibitors are the first-line treatment, followed by beta blockers and thiazides, then calcium channel antagonists. Once-daily preparations are more likely to be remembered than multiple-dosage regimens. Obviously, all blood pressure lowering agents are capable of causing hypotension—particularly postural hypotension—which may be worse in patients with autonomic neuropathy. This should be sought by asking about postural dizziness or light-headedness, and by measuring lying and standing blood pressures. ACE inhibitors, beta blockers, and diuretics can all cause fluid or electrolyte imbalance. Many hypotensive agents interact with other drugs and this should be checked before prescribing. They can cause erectile dysfunction.

ACE inhibitors

Captopril, enalapril, fosinopril, lisinopril, and ramipril have all been shown to be effective in people with diabetes. In addition to lowering blood pressure some ACE inhibitors are known to reduce urinary protein leak, and lisinopril can reduce retinopathy. Ramipril reduces cardiac events and stroke. First-dose hypotension varies with different agents but is more likely in fluid-depleted patients such as those on diuretics. ACE inhibitors can cause renal failure in patients with renal artery stenosis so should be used with caution in arteriopaths. Check urea and electrolytes pre-treatment, and regularly on treatment. ACE inhibitors can cause high plasma potassium levels. They often cause chronic dry cough, and may produce taste disturbances, rashes, and, rarely, marrow suppression. Patients with aortic stenosis should usually avoid ACE inhibitors. They may cause foetal malformation, so women of child-bearing potential should use reliable contraception—or another antihypertensive. Angioedema can occur.

ACE II inhibitors

Have also been shown to be of benefit in diabetes. They can be substituted if the cough is troublesome with ACE inhibitors.

Beta blockers

Atenolol was shown to be safe and effective in UKPDS (see p. 29). Beta blockers reduce warning of hypoglycaemia—tell patients of this, especially those on insulin. Avoid in patients with asthma or chronic obstructive pulmonary disease, with brady-cardia or heart block, with uncompensated heart failure, and severe peripheral vascular disease. Beta blockers may cause exertional tiredness, cold extremities, sleep disturbance, and bradycardia.

Diuretics

Bendrofluazide and hydrochlorothiazide have both been shown to be safe and effective in diabetes. Thiazides were used in UKPDS (see p. 29). Although they may increase blood glucose this was not a problem, nor was electrolyte disturbance. Urea and electrolytes should be measured pre-treatment and regularly thereafter. Diuretics combined with beta blockers seem particularly likely to cause hypokalaemia in clinical practice. 2.5 mg bendrofluazide is sufficient to achieve a hypotensive effect. Thiazides should be used with care in pregnancy (and only in a specialist centre).

Calcium channel antagonists

Amlodipine, felodipine, nifedipine (long-acting), and others. It has been suggested that calcium channel antagonists may increase the risk of cardiac events in people with diabetes. However, most studies have not confirmed this. There are several different types of calcium channel, and different drugs affect different channels, with varying side-effects. Calcium channel antagonists do not cause fluid, electrolyte, or glucose changes. They do cause vasodilatation, and this may cause headache, flushing, or ankle swelling. Class II agents (such as those above) are less likely to depress cardiac contraction than Class I agents such as verapamil. These drugs should be avoided in pregnancy.

Young diabetic women with hypertension

Most hypotensive agents are contraindicated in pregnancy. Diabetic women not planning pregnancy should use reliable contraception while taking hypotensive drugs. Increasingly, women with diabetic complications, including hypertension, are planning pregnancy. Such women should use methyl dopa with careful monitoring until they have completed their family. They should be referred for specialist peri-pregnancy diabetes care.

Peripheral vascular disease

After 20 years of diabetes, half the men and two-thirds of the women over 60 years old have no foot pulses. People with diabetes are two to four times as likely to experience intermittent claudication as non-diabetics, and four to six times as likely to have an amputation. Up to 50 per cent of people requiring amputation have diabetes.

Screening—peripheral vascular disease

- Screen all patients on diagnosis and annually thereafter.
- Check smoking history. Ask about intermittent claudication.
- Look at the feet for evidence of ischaemia and feel the dorsalis pedis and posterior tibial pulses.
- Measure cholesterol and triglyceride (see p. 136).

Assessment of peripheral vascular disease

Patients may have calf or buttock pain. If the patient has symptoms or absent pulses, check with a Doppler probe if you have one. Palpate the popliteal and femoral pulses and listen for femoral bruits.

Warning signs

- Gradually worsening symptoms. Refer the patient to a vascular surgeon.
- Rest pain. Telephone the diabetologist or vascular surgeon to arrange an admission under their joint care.
- Critical ischaemia—red, painful. Poor capillary refilling.
- Acute ischaemia—white/blue; cold, pulseless, painful foot/limb. Transfer to hospital immediately to be seen by the vascular and diabetes teams.
- Gangrene. Transfer to hospital immediately to be seen by the vascular and diabetes team.
- Any foot problem in addition to the peripheral vascular disease (see p. 146)

Treatment of peripheral vascular disease

Insist that the patient stops smoking and vigorously support his efforts to do so. Encourage exercise (take care this does not exacerbate other foot problems such as pressure areas). Encourage a low-fat diet and control hyperlipidaemia if present. Stop

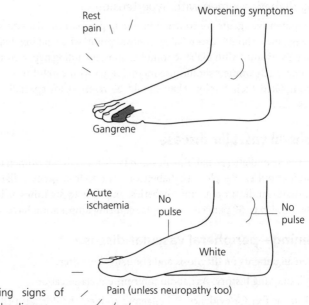

Rest pain

Worsening symptoms

Gangrene

Acute ischaemia

No pulse

No pulse

White

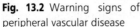

Fig. 13.2 Warning signs of peripheral vascular disease

Pain (unless neuropathy too)

beta blockers. Naftidrofuryl oxalate (Praxilene) may relieve symptoms but it should be remembered that resolution can occur spontaneously as collaterals open up.

The consequences of peripheral vascular disease are disastrous and all patients should be assessed jointly by a vascular surgeon and diabetologist. Angiography is performed in patients with worsening symptoms or whose limb is at risk and who would be suitable for surgery. It usually reveals multiple stenoses with diffuse distal disease. Angioplasty is sometimes possible and both proximal and distal arterial bypass are being used increasingly. Amputation is discussed on p. 150.

Summary

- Diabetic tissue damage can blind, cripple, and kill. It can be prevented.
- Patients and diabetes carers must make strenuous efforts to prevent diabetes tissue damage.
- Patient education is a vital factor in helping patients to reduce their risk of tissue damage.
- To reduce the risk of tissue damage people with diabetes should:
  keep their blood pressure normal;
  keep their blood glucose levels as near normal as is safe;
  keep their blood lipids normal;
  keep their weight normal;
  not smoke;
  exercise regularly.

• To detect tissue damage early, screen eyes, kidneys, nerve function, feet, and cardiovascular system at least annually.

References and further reading

Ariffin, A., Hill, R.D. and Leigh, O. (1992). Diabetes and Primary Eye Care. Blackwell Scientific Publications. Oxford.

Cavallerano, J.D. (1990). A review of non-retinal ocular complications of diabetes mellitus. *J. Am. Optom. Assoc.*, **61**, 533–43.

DCCT Research Group (1993). The effect of intensive treatment of diabetes on the development and progression of long-term complications of IDDM. *New England Journal of Medicine*, **329**, 977–86.

Department of Health (2000). *National service frameworks for coronary heart disease*. HMSO.

Kritzinger, E. and Taylor, K. (1984). *Diabetic eye disease*. Kluwer Academic Publishers, Lancaster.

Chapter 14

The diabetic foot

Diabetic foot problems are largely preventable. Assal *et al.* (1982) dramatically reduced the amputation rate in a Swiss diabetes service by introducing an intensive patient education and foot care programme.

Why are the feet so vulnerable?

We bear our entire weight on our feet, subjecting their components to enormous stresses every day. Early warning of problems helps us to protect our feet.

Neuropathy

Diabetic neuropathy reduces sensation of pain, touch, temperature, and position. Rubs, scrapes, and knocks are ignored because they cannot be felt. Patients may walk around with a pebble in their shoe all day without realizing. Skin may be burned by near-boiling water with no sensation of heat or pain. If you do not know where your foot is in space, you cannot keep it in the best position for weight-bearing safely. Callus can build up under the metatarsal heads and elsewhere. Neuropathy may alter the circulation, causing arteriovenous shunting and depriving tissues of oxygen.

Microvascular disease

Small vessel disease may damage the healing response, so that minor injuries are not repaired and infections may eventually spread to threaten the viability of deeper tissues.

Vascular disease

Atheroma is common in diabetes, affecting not only large vessels but smaller ones, for example those supplying the legs and feet in which calcification may be seen on X-ray. Poor circulation causes symptoms of its own—intermittent claudication, rest pain, and finally gangrene. In addition it worsens other problems by depriving injured or infected areas of oxygen, slowing healing, and allowing anaerobic bacteria to flourish. Antibiotics may not reach the areas of infection in sufficient concentrations to be effective.

Deformity

Diabetes can cause ligamentous changes. In the feet this may lead to clawed or hammer toes. This causes further abnormalities of weight bearing, and the curled toes may get corns on top as they rub against shoes. Neuropathy, vasculopathy, and infection may cause damage leading to deformity, as can surgery. The foot then develops multiple pressure points and callus builds up.

Bones

Bone density is reduced in people with diabetes, more so in those with Type 1, than in Type 2. Diabetic autonomic neuropathy intensifies this process in the feet with increased vascularity and shunting. When this is combined with peripheral neuropathy, small injuries can initiate bony destruction and distortion, which extends rapidly with continued weight bearing or repeated injury. The bones and joints are gradually destroyed causing Charcot joints.

Infection

Hyperglycaemia reduces white cell mobility and a poor blood supply slows delivery of white cells and nutrients, thereby impeding the body's defensive response to infection. Via areas of callus, pockets of infection can extend deep into the foot and thence into the tissue planes. Infections there and elsewhere do not hurt and progress rapidly.

Other problems

If they cannot feel pain, even those who can see or smell a problem may not treat it with the seriousness it deserves: 'If it doesn't hurt it can't be too bad'. 'It can't be happening to me.' Those who are aware of the seriousness may be so frightened of losing their foot or leg that they conceal the problems. Partially sighted patients may not be able to see trouble developing on their feet.

> Marion was a 60-year-old woman with long-standing Type 1 diabetes. She attended diabetic clinic between annual reviews. 'Are your feet all right?' asked the doctor. 'Yes, thank you,' she replied. Three weeks later she was admitted with infected gangrene of her toe. At that point she confessed that she had gangrene at the time of her clinic visit but had been so terrified of being admitted to hospital that she had lied to her doctor. The infection spread, despite vigorous antibiotic and other treatment. Her leg was amputated. She developed a chest infection. Her condition deteriorated and she finally died from a massive myocardial infarct after many months as an in-patient.

Prevention of diabetic foot problems

There are two facets to this—patient education and staff education. Many people know that diabetes can lead to leg amputation. But patients may still fail to take the practical steps to prevent themselves ending up in a wheelchair too. Health care professionals, whether in hospital or in general practice, fail to take the time to check patients' feet themselves and often fail to act sufficiently vigorously when patients present with what look like minor foot problems. A small blister on a little toe can lead to amputation.

Guidelines for doctors

Examine every diabetic patient's feet on diagnosis and annually. On examination check:

- Skin—colour, ulcers, rubs, blisters, corns, calluses, etc.
- Foot and toe shape—hammer or claw toes, bunions, missing toes, surgery, deformities

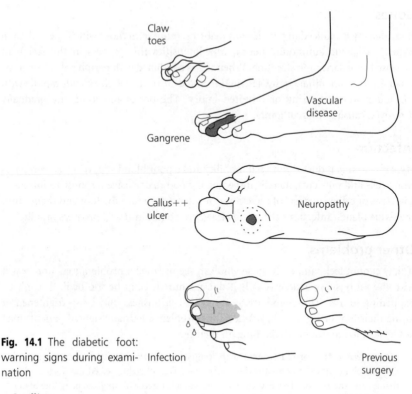

Fig. 14.1 The diabetic foot: warning signs during examination

- Swelling
- Pulses—dorsalis pedis and posterior tibial
- Sensation—light touch, Monofilament, vibration, position
- Hygiene
- Shoes and hosiery.

Danger signs

Colour change Red foot (infection or 'sunset' ischaemic foot); white (no circulation); blue/black (gangrene). Refer to hospital immediately.

Infection Any foot infection in patients with neuropathy or vascular disease should be treated by staff used to such problems. This is usually the hospital diabetes team. If you suspect any infection is major or extends below the immediate subcutaneous tissues refer the patient to hospital immediately. Superficial infected areas should be cleaned and dressed (see Table 14.1) and seen daily by a nurse or doctor until healed. Any infection which is not healing within three days should be referred to hospital. Refer patients with worsening foot or leg infection to hospital immediately.

Swelling This may mean infection, autonomic neuropathy, Charcot joints, cardiac failure, or nephrotic syndrome. It is often a danger sign in people with diabetes. Consider referral to a diabetologist.

Table 14.1 Look after your feet: guidelines for patients

1. Look at your feet every day. Use a mirror or ask someone else to help if you have difficulty seeing.

2. If you have any of the following see your doctor (or chiropodist or diabetic clinic) within 24 hours:

   any colour change

   any new pain or unusual feeling

   any sore places (corns, blisters, cracks, calluses, ulcers, bunions)

   swelling anywhere

   any break in the skin (ulcers, cracks, blisters)

   a strange smell from your feet

3. Treat any skin break by washing with dilute antiseptic (follow the instructions on the container), drying gently with sterile gauze, and covering with a dry dressing (e.g. N-A dressing). Use non-allergic tape (e.g. Micropore) and **never** wind it round a toe. Then contact help.

4. Wash your feet daily in lukewarm water. Dry carefully, especially between the toes.

5. If you have dry skin use a moisturizing cream or emollient lotion, but not between the toes.

6. Cut toenails in a gentle curve without leaving sharp edges to dig in to that or other toes.

7. Wear clean socks, stockings, or tights every day.

8. Buy shoes which do not squeeze your foot, and which do not hurt or rub anywhere the first time you try them on. Low-heeled lace-ups with plenty of toe room are best.

9. Do not walk bare foot.

10. Do not use corn cures, or cut corns or callus.

11. Do not use a hot water bottle.

12. Do not use vibrating foot massagers or baths.

13. Do not smoke.

14. See a state registered chiropodist regularly (SRCh).

This table may be photocopied for use by patients only. ©2002 Dr Rowan Hillson. From *Practical diabetes care*, Oxford University Press, 2002.

Pain This requires urgent investigation. It may represent an easily treatable problem, tight shoes for example. Or it may represent major trouble such as infection. Remember that neuropathy may blunt pain but that it can also cause pain. Furthermore, although Charcot joints develop in neuropathic limbs, they may be painful while evolving. Repeat X-rays in diabetic neuropathic patients with persistent pain, swelling, or heat after an injury.

Heat A hot area may indicate infection or an active Charcot joint. Such 'hot spots' should always be investigated.

Cold A cold foot or leg strongly suggests vascular insufficiency. Rapidly developing coldness indicates acute vascular block and the need for urgent action (see p. 143).

Absent foot pulses (See p. 143).

Neuropathy (See p. 131).

Who should treat foot problems?

Any patient with a foot problem is at risk of further trouble and it is sensible to examine their feet whenever you see them (a) to reinforce the message of foot care to patients and (b) to spot early trouble. All diabetic patients should have priority access to chiropody and those with any foot problem should have regular chiropody.

The best place to treat such patients is at a diabetes foot clinic where all the relevant specialists see the patient together. If this is not available the diabetes team are likely to have the most experience of dealing with such problems and it is usually best to refer foot emergencies directly to the diabetes service. Check your local arrangements before you need them. The diabetologist will then co-ordinate all care with vascular surgery, orthopaedics, chiropody, wound care, special shoes, rehabilitation, and so on. It is vital that good communication is maintained with the general practitioner and that he is fully informed of the details of the discharge care plan. After discharge the general practitioner must make sure that all facets of care are actually happening— gaps are common due to lapses in communication or transport failures. One missed treatment may be disastrous.

Amputation

Around half the amputees in Britain have diabetes. Amputation is one of the most feared complications of diabetes. When investigating the pathway leading to amputa- tion one can often chart a succession of small practical problems and unfortunate coincidences. The ambulance did not come so the patient missed her clinic appoint- ment. The out-patient computer re-booked a three-month appointment for the one which the patient failed to attend. The district nurse was in a hurry so the patient did not like to trouble her about the foot ulcer. The patient could not get an appointment with her general practitioner until next week and the ulcer did not hurt so it hardly seemed urgent. And so on.

Patients requiring amputation will often have been in hospital for many weeks or months. The loss of a leg can produce a bereavement reaction as profound as that of losing a close relative. The patient needs a lot of support, especially when they are discharged from hospital. They have been cared for by nurses and other staff in a secure environment; suddenly they are at home discovering that many of the things they used to be able to do are no longer easy or possible.

The stage at which the patient has been discharged will vary slightly. The stump will probably be healed and they may be using a stump sock to keep it in shape. The patient will have had sessions with the occupational therapist and physiotherapist and will probably still be attending out-patient visits. At first patients begin to learn how to walk using an inflatable support on the stump. They will also have been taught how to use crutches and/or a frame and a wheelchair and how to transfer. In many cases care will be co-ordinated by a physician in rehabilitation medicine who will see the patient before the operation, while they are in hospital, and afterwards at the limb fitting centre. Once the stump is healed the patient will be measured for an artificial limb. It is important that patients realize that this takes time to make and that there may have to be several fittings before they can walk on it. Patients can become frustrated at this stage. Stump problems are common in patients with diabetes and a close eye should be kept on its condition. It is also crucial to protect the other foot and leg (see p. 149). Half of all diabetic amputees die or lose their other leg within 3 years.

Although the patient's attention is often focused on the leg and arrangements for walking again, attention must also be paid to other facets of their life. Blood glucose control is important for good healing. Hypoglycaemia is common as the physiotherapy progresses and must be avoided at home as the patient may find it hard to cope with. The patient often has other problems such as cardiac or renal disease and may have retinopathy. Practical aspects of home care such as urine bottles, a commode, where they are going to sleep, preparing meals, coping with domestic crises, keeping warm, must all be sorted out. A telephone is essential, and a portable phone which can be carried in a wheelchair or moved from room to room, is best. The patient's housing may be unsuitable (e.g. have very steep stairs). Consider a move if the problem cannot be remedied.

Patients worry about finances and about returning to work. Patients working for employers are eligible for statutory sick pay for up to 28 weeks followed by invalidity benefit, but self-employed patients may be in severe financial difficulties. The patient will need a sheaf of paperwork supported by his doctor. Each amputee should have a social worker to help him through the complexities and ensure that he does obtain all his allowances. Relatives caring for him may also attract allowances and tax reductions. If the patient has a sedentary job they can usually return early. Those with active jobs may have to change them although many amputees return to a completely normal life and normal activities. The problem for people with diabetes may be that they are older than traumatic amputees (e.g. servicemen injured in war) and that they have other problems with rehabilitation such as neuropathy in their remaining leg. Patients can register disabled for employment purposes and may then get appropriate posts as part of the quota scheme.

When so many personnel are involved in a patient's care and rehabilitation there may be wasteful duplication; alternatively the patient can fall between two stools. The GP should be the central co-ordinator of care and it is helpful to keep an action plan and contact numbers of those involved with the patient's care in their records. The action plan should be reviewed regularly with the patient and his family.

Summary

- Diabetes foot problems are preventable
- The consequence may be amputation
- Educate the patient about daily foot care
- Take a personal interest in their feet; check at least annually
- Examine high-risk feet at every visit
- Respond urgently to any foot problems. An ulcer this big ● may eventually kill the patient.

References

Assal, J.-Ph., Gfeller, R., and Ekoe, J.M. (1982). Patient education in diabetes. In *Recent trends in diabetes research* (ed. H. Bostrom), pp. 276–90. Almquist & Wiksell International, Stockholm.

NICE (2002). Management of Type 2 diabetes. Renal disease - prevention and early management. Inherited Clinical Guideline F. *www.nice.org.uk*

NICE (2002). Management of Type 2 diabetes. Retinopathy - screening and early management. Inherited Clinical Guideline E. *www.nice.org.uk*

Royal College of General Practitioners Effective Clinical Practice Unit, University of Sheffield. Clinical Guidelines for Type 2 Diabetes. Diabetic retinopathy: early management and screening (2002). *www.nice.org.uk*

Chapter 15

Growing up with diabetes

Young people with diabetes are often challenging to care for and they need specialized diabetes care, preferably under joint supervision by a paediatrician and a diabetologist. Their diabetes will be affected by, or will influence most other health care issues. The GP's special knowledge of the young person's family situation makes him a valuable member of the care team. Diabetes may also have a major effect upon the young person's parents and siblings—and vice versa. Communication between the services (often many) involved must remain good at all times.

Presentation of diabetes in children

The majority of diabetic children will be insulin-dependent. However, Type 2 diabetes is found sometimes—especially in overweight teenagers. Diabetes presents with the same symptoms as in adults. Additional features may include growth retardation, difficulties at school, behavioural problems, and bed-wetting or regression from toilet training. The symptoms may be difficult to discern in very small children in whom urine (preferably blood) glucose screening should form part of general assessment in illness.

Treatment of diabetes in children

Many children now start insulin treatment at home without hospital admission, although some centres still admit the child and a parent for a few days initially. The home start approach can be achieved only by a dedicated diabetologist/paediatrician who provides personal care, or by a diabetes specialist nurse (preferably paediatrically trained). Other members of the team may be seen at the hospital or at home. The child and their family are visited once or twice a day until they are confident in insulin injection technique and diet. A 24-hour telephone diabetes help-line is essential in this situation.

Children should have two injections a day, or four if using short-acting insulin before meals. Good blood glucose balance can rarely be achieved on once-daily insulin. They and their parents need to be warned about the honeymoon period of diabetes in which the last remaining beta cells, released from the effects of hyperglycaemia, produce some insulin before succumbing to the continuing autoimmune destructive process. Insulin requirements may fall to one or two units for a few weeks or months, before rising again. Pre-warning is essential to avoid bitter disappointment—'I thought my diabetes had gone away'. (Adults with Type 1 diabetes may experience the honeymoon period too.)

Complications start in childhood

It used to be said that only diabetes after puberty 'counted' towards the development of diabetic tissue damage. This is untrue. In fact, children as young as 10 years old can develop retinopathy. Patients whose Type 1 diabetes began in childhood are much more likely to have proteinuria than those diagnosed as adults but with similar duration (Allagoa *et al.* 2001). We have to improve diabetes care in children and teenagers—failure to do so may seriously impair quality and quantity of life.

Practical difficulties

Listen to the child. If he has a problem it can often be resolved by attention to detail or by changing the technology. In a world in which the child perceives the doctor as a headmaster-like figure, the diabetes specialist nurse or practice nurse may be more likely to find out what the real problem is.

Injections

No one likes injections but children are sometimes less upset about them than their parents anticipate. Parents (both mother and father) should always learn how to give the injections but if at all possible the child should start by giving their own injections. There is no need to use an alcohol swab and it hurts more. Insulin pens make this easier and their needles appear to hurt less (perhaps because they do not also pierce the insulin bottle bung). However, the pen may be too big for the child to manage. Perpendicular injections, although easier, may cause intramuscular injection. 'Pinch and prick' techniques are better.

Finger-prick glucose tests

Often finger-prick blood tests are more unpopular with the child than the insulin injections. Great care should be taken to find the finger-pricking system and part of finger which hurts least. Safety tests (before bed, before sport, when ill) are the ones which should be insisted upon, although ideally the tests should be more frequent to allow insulin and dietary adjustment.

Diet

> Carol was a 22-year-old medical student. She had had diabetes since she was 5 years old. Her parents and her doctor had thought it cruel to make her stick to a nasty diabetic diet and she had been allowed to eat what she wanted provided she had her injections. She now had diabetic retinopathy and renal damage and bitterly resented the years of lax diabetes control. She particularly resented never having been given the chance to decide between compliance or not.

Food is the commonest battleground between the diabetic child and his or her parents. This is hardly surprising as all children use food as a weapon. The diabetic diet is the healthy diet which everyone should follow and it helps if the whole family has the same diet. Some sugar can be included as part of meals and this approach may be more likely to gain general dietary compliance than banning sweets altogether, although some paediatricians would disagree with this. The child must eat enough to grow properly—the 'diet' must not be interpreted as weight restricting unless the child is actually obese. There is no place for 'diabetic' foods and fatty foods should be discouraged. Introduce the new diet gradually and help the child to learn about different types of food and how they might affect diabetes.

Battles

Diabetes is a very effective weapon. A sulking, non-diabetic child who refuses to eat can be told 'If you don't eat it you will go without.' The diabetic child knows that once the insulin has been injected, his parents will be desperate for him to eat to avoid hypoglycaemia. He also knows that refusing an insulin injection will get his parents really worked up. There is no easy solution—it is simple for the outsider to say 'Don't let it become an issue'—they do not have to live with the child and his diabetes every day. Nowadays, ultrafast insulins such as insulin lispro or aspart can be given after eating, although more experience of their use in children is needed. One approach may be to help parents and children learn how flexible they can be with diabetes care—to explore their limits. Many parents are so frightened of possible adverse consequences that they adhere rigidly to the guidelines they were given on diagnosis without realizing that some flexibility is possible. Many need a lot of support in introducing flexibility. There are limits for all aspects of care and a balance must be struck between flexibility and *laissez faire*.

> A group of young teenagers with diabetes went on a mountain walk. It took longer than everyone expected. By their usual evening mealtime they were still high on the mountain. So they had a large snack, and some had insulin according to their usual regimen and their current blood glucose. By the time they returned to base it was three hours past their mealtime. None had major problems with their blood glucose. In a review session they angrily accused staff, 'You made us late for supper, diabetics must never be late for a meal'. 'You're all right, aren't you', I replied. Long pause for thought 'Yes, we are, aren't we.' We then discussed ways of coping with a late meal or a late injection.

Growth

Sadly, 'diabetic dwarfs' still exist. These young people have had high blood glucose levels during the time when they would otherwise have been growing. Insulin deficiency has profound effects on growth and development because hyperglycaemia suppresses growth hormone release. Normoglycaemia with a healthy diet containing sufficient calories is essential for normal growth. All diabetic young people under the age of 19 should have a growth chart (height and weight) in their hospital and GP records. Mark their parents' heights on the chart too. If any slowing of growth is observed, prompt action is required to elucidate the cause and treat it or it may be too late.

Puberty

Puberty, with its changing hormonal balance and metabolic demands, is usually a time when insulin dose increases and when blood glucose balance may become erratic. Menstruation can cause cyclical hyperglycaemia (sometimes hypoglycaemia). Do not increase the insulin so much that the young person needs to eat more and becomes overweight. However, food intake usually increases around puberty. Diabetic girls who have started to menstruate must be told about sexual intercourse, the possibility of pregnancy, and the need for family planning in diabetes. With the recent AIDS prevention campaigns, and ready availability of condoms in shops, sexual ignorance is less common than before. An unsuspected pregnancy can precipitate diabetic keto-acidosis and it is particularly important to avoid unwanted pregnancy in diabetic girls.

Adolescence

One diabetic young woman can amass ten volumes of hospital notes, and engage the attentions of the diabetes team, all the on-take medical teams in the hospital, the social services, the GP, and practice staff. Her parents may require psychiatric and medical help, and some staff may need psychological support. However, although the dramatic behaviour of the 'brittle diabetic' is often memorable and time-consuming, remember that there are only one or two such patients in most districts.

Adolescence is a time of experimentation with one's personality, one's sexuality, one's family, and the outside world. In our society it is often 'make or break' time—exam results determine further training, apprenticeships further careers, marriage partners may be chosen. It is a time when young people test their boundaries such as their parents' authority, school or college rules, their health and fitness, relationships with others. It is also a time when parents must start handing over diabetes care to their children, if they have not already done so. This can be very difficult. The worries of a parent waiting for a child to come home from a late night disco are compounded when that child has diabetes. Has she eaten enough? Will she drink too much? If she is late, has she gone hypo? It is hard to relinquish care of a potentially dangerous disorder at the very time when a young person is rebelling against authority and appears least capable of taking care of themselves.

Young people with diabetes between the ages of about 15 and 25 years should be seen in a young persons' diabetic clinic by a team experienced in their care. The transfer from the children's diabetic clinic occurs when the young person is ready to do so. Some young people do not wish to attend any hospital clinic and for them the GP is the key carer. The GP is in a good position to insist on seeing the young person regularly—he prescribes the insulin. The first aim is for the professional of the young person's choice to maintain contact. The next is to ensure regular insulin injections, then dietary compliance and blood testing with appropriate treatment adjustment. A judgemental authoritarian approach is rarely successful and merely alienates the young person. Listen to what the patient says and make sure he knows that his opinion is heard and respected. It may take many months or years to build up a clinical relationship with a young person during this vulnerable phase of their diabetic life. If the worst happens and contact is lost, try at least to ensure that the young person knows exactly where to come for help when he is ill or in trouble. If the 'lost sheep' returns, welcome them, deal with any emergencies swiftly, then apply a constructive approach to future improvements in care.

Areas for patient education during adolescence include eating (including discussion of junk foods), alcohol, school, further education and work, sex, and discussion of the long-term effects of diabetes on the body. There is nothing to be gained from hiding the complications of diabetes from a young person. They will all be aware of some of them, and will usually have an unduly black picture. New diabetes technology, for example biosensors and insulin pens may be particularly attractive to young people and their convenience and 'street credibility' may improve compliance.

Education and diabetes

Diabetes UK provides an excellent schools pack which is essential reading for parents and teachers of diabetic children. Most large schools will have one or two children with diabetes. Areas of self care which can make diabetes easier to manage at school are dietary knowledge, blood glucose testing, awareness of the symptoms of hypo-glycaemia and how to treat them, and knowledge of how to cope with exercise. Self injection means that the child can go on school trips, too. It is best for the child that everyone (including fellow pupils) is aware that he or she has diabetes—otherwise there may be unpleasant accusations of drug abuse if injections or blood tests are observed.

There is rarely any need for a diabetic child to take time off school and repeated school absences because of diabetes must be investigated promptly so that diabetes care can be improved. There is a complex interrelationship between poor glycaemic balance, the psychological effects of diabetes, school work, and behaviour. Resolution may require the combined efforts of a parents, teachers, child psychologist, paediatri-cian, diabetes team, and GP; clear communication is vital. Most diabetic children do as well as their non-diabetic peers academically, and there is some suggestion that they may do better, perhaps because of greater pressure to succeed.

> Ann developed diabetes just before she was due to take up a hard-won place at university. She felt that she would not be able to cope with both diabetes and university and gave up her place.

The development of diabetes can ruin a university or college career, or other training. This is an unnecessary tragedy as most young people complete their train-ing unimpeded by their diabetes. Prompt diagnosis and treatment focused on a return to academic or practical activities as soon as possible can minimize the dam-age. However, in some instances, the young person may be unable to perform up to their usual standard for a few weeks or occasionally months. The doctor may be able to explain to academic or training authorities and help the patient to gain another chance.

For a young person who wishes to be completely flexible and who enjoys life on the move, an easily portable diabetes kit includes an insulin pen for thrice-daily fast-acting insulin (the night-time long-acting or intermediate-acting insulin can be left at home), a compact meter for glucose measurement, some readily portable snacks, dextrosol, and a diabetic card.

Summary

- Children usually have Type 1 diabetes.
- Diabetes in small children and young people requires specialist care.
- Near normoglycaemia is essential for normal growth and development.
- Try not to allow diabetes care to become a war zone between parents and children.
- Help young people and their parents to develop safe, flexible diabetes care.
- Maintain contact with diabetic adolescents. Teach them about their diabetes and provide non-judgemental support.
- Listen to what the patient says.

Reference

Allagoa, B. *et al.* (2001). The influence of age at onset of Type 1 diabetes on the development of diabetic nephropathy. *Diabetic Medicine*, **18** (suppl. 2), 35.

Chapter 16

The family and the diabetic man or woman

Diabetes in one family member influences all the others, indeed, some family members may subsequently develop diabetes themselves. It is important that family and friends realize that diabetes is not infectious. The risk of inheriting diabetes differs between Type 1 and Type 2, and is difficult to quantify as the development of diabetes appears to be an amalgam of genetics and environment. Published estimations vary.

Inheritance of diabetes

Type 1 diabetes

An identical twin has a 30–50 per cent chance of developing Type 1 diabetes if his twin has it. The sibling of someone with Type 1 diabetes has about an 8 per cent chance of developing diabetes (this can be better predicted if HLA typing is done, but this is not performed outside research projects). A child has a 1–2 per cent chance of developing diabetes if his mother has it and a 6 per cent chance if his father has it. If both parents have Type 1 diabetes, the risk is 30 per cent. These figures should be compared with the frequency of Type 1 diabetes in the population as a whole which is 0.25 per cent and rising.

Type 2 diabetes

The chance of inheriting Type 2 diabetes is harder to assess as some individuals do not develop the disease until their 80s. There is virtually 100 per cent concordance of diabetes in identical twins. About 25 per cent of the relatives of someone with Type 2 diabetes have had, have, or eventually develop diabetes. If one parent has Type 2 diabetes about 15 per cent of their children will eventually develop it; if both parents have Type 2 diabetes the risk may be as high as 75 per cent. The frequency in the population as a whole is 2–3 per cent and rising.

The impact of diabetes upon the family

The discovery of diabetes in a child can cause major stresses within a family. If a parent has it, there may be much self-blame. The pattern of family life may be interrupted by the mechanics of diabetes care. Other siblings may feel left out as much attention and anxiety is lavished upon their brother or sister. They may also be frightened, especially if their sibling was rushed to hospital very ill. 'Is Johnny going to die? Am I going to catch diabetes?'

If an adult develops diabetes the impact upon the family is variable. Some self-sufficient couples cope well:

> Alexander developed diabetes days before his wife was due to deliver their first child. Within three days the couple had bought a selection of diabetes books, learned how to master his treatment and blood testing, and had the satisfaction of seeing his blood glucose begin to fall. By the time the child was born Alexander's blood glucose was normal and both parents became fully occupied in caring for their baby daughter.

Others react differently:

> Ernest was horrified when his wife developed diabetes. The elderly couple had experienced no serious illnesses before. He took over her diet, her treatment, and even talked for her during consultations. Doris appeared to know nothing about her diabetes and the diabetes team were never able to persuade her to take any interest in her condition. When Doris developed an infection her husband tried to manage her diabetes alone at home for some days and she was seriously ill and grossly hyperglycaemic when she was finally admitted. Ernest spend every day in hospital with her. He became exhausted and finally confessed that he was having chest pain. He was admitted and it was some weeks before both were fit enough for discharge.

In some families the diabetes diet is seen as very unusual. The person with diabetes may have to sit watching everyone else eat bacon, sausage, and chips followed by chocolate whip and sugary biscuits while she eats chicken salad and fruit. Women are more likely to change their diet to a diabetes one if their husband has diabetes than vice versa. As the diabetes diet is that recommended for the population at large the whole family should adopt it.

Diabetes may become an open, accepted part of family life, a weapon or defence, or an enemy which causes disability or financial disaster. The person with diabetes needs the full support of his or her family. If the patient agrees, close family members should be encouraged to meet the diabetes team and learn more about diabetes. The GP and practice team can provide diabetes education, and support family members as well as the patient.

Home circumstances

For optimal care, it is essential that people with diabetes live in accommodation in which they can readily maintain a high standard of personal hygiene, where they can keep their medication and equipment secure and where they are not exposed to extremes of temperature, or infection due, for example, to poor food storage or infestation. Every person with diabetes must have a telephone or be able to summon help if taken ill at home, 24 hours a day. If financial difficulties are endangering the person's health and well-being, Diabetes UK can provide information about charitable funds.

Women

All the changes of womanhood can influence, and be influenced by, diabetes.

Menstruation

The hormonal changes preceding and during menstruation can cause both hypo-glycaemia and hyperglycaemia in different individuals. The most frequent change is hyperglycaemia, on the last day or so premenstrually or, most often, during the first two days of bleeding. Some women are hypoglycaemic premenstrually or as the bleeding subsides. In others unpredictable oscillations in glycaemic balance appear to be the problem. Some women increase their insulin for the first two days of bleeding. Hyperglycaemia can cause menstrual irregularity or amenorrhoea, especially in untreated diabetes.

Infections

Vaginal thrush is a common presenting feature in diabetic women and is often dif-ficult to eradicate. The perineal soreness and irritation can be extremely distressing and may cause irritability and sleep disturbance. Good glycaemic control improves the chances of cure using standard antifungals. The partner should be treated as well. Herpes simplex and herpes zoster, and vaginal warts all appear more common in women with diabetes. Urinary tract infections can add to the woman's misery and it may co-exist with candidiasis.

Contraception

Barrier methods, preferably sheath and spermicide, are the best option, but only if properly used. Condoms protect both partners from infection, protect the cervix from sperm and have no effect on blood glucose. They are also easily bought in a wide variety of shops, supermarkets, and garages. A diaphragm requires gynaecological assessment for fitting and there may be an increased risk of vaginal and urinary infec-tion. However, barrier methods are useless if not used properly; planned conception and the avoidance of unwanted pregnancy are particularly important in women with diabetes.

Intra-uterine contraceptive devices (IUCDs) are rarely used in nulliparous women. In any woman there is a risk of pelvic infection rarely leading to infertility. This risk is greater in women with diabetes because of their propensity to infection generally. Older forms of IUCD underwent unusual chemical change in some women with dia-betes and failed to prevent conception. This does not appear to be a problem with currently used IUCDs.

Oral contraceptive pills are the most effective form of contraception but they impair glucose tolerance and cause lipid abnormalities, both of which are already a problem in women with diabetes. The risk of cardiovascular and thromboembolic complica-tions is undesirable as diabetes already predisposes to the former, if not the latter. Hypertension also occurs in both Pill use and diabetes. A woman with diabetes and her partner are therefore encouraged to use barrier contraception if possible. How-ever, many couples do not wish to use barrier methods or cannot use them effectively. Many diabetologists would advise progestogen-only preparations (initially, changing to a combined oestrogen/progestogen preparation) if the progestogen-only preparation is not acceptable. The patient's glucose balance, lipids, and blood pressure must be monitored regularly.

The rhythm method and withdrawal are not effective and cannot be recommended for diabetic women.

Post-coital contraception using levonorgestrol and ethinyloestradiol can be initiated within 72 hours of unprotected intercourse.

Pre-pregnancy counselling

Diabetic women have near-normal fertility unless they have persistently high blood glucose levels, or have renal impairment. Even then, conception can occur. Teenage girls should know that it is important to plan pregnancy when they do decide to have a family and that contraception should be used, if necessary, until then.

Congenital malformations used to be two to three times as common in diabetic pregnancies as in the general population. Then it was found that malformations were most likely in women with hyperglycaemia in the first 8 weeks of pregnancy, (for example women whose haemoglobin $A1_c$ was over 10 per cent). Maintenance of strict normoglycaemia reduces the likelihood of congenital malformation to near that of the non-diabetic population.

As few women know when they conceive, the usual strategy is to maintain contraception, adjust treatment to achieve normoglycaemia, and then stop the contraception. It is easier to use barrier methods here, as menstrual cycles may be erratic after stopping oral contraception and it is helpful to be able to date the last menstrual period if pregnancy occurs. Normoglycaemia is continued. It is hard work and means four times daily finger-prick glucose estimations, sometimes for years if conception is slow to occur.

Few women of child-bearing age will be taking oral hypoglycaemic drugs. This is more common in women of Asian and Afro-Caribbean origin. There is concern that these drugs may be associated with fetal malformation. Stop them and transfer the patient to insulin treatment.

The woman's fitness to withstand pregnancy and her prospects of healthy survival during the years in which her child needs her most must also be considered. Nowadays, women with severe tissue damage are surviving pregnancy with normal infants, but this requires nine months very intensive effort, and the harsh reality is that they may become severely disabled or die before their child grows up. Retinopathy can worsen in pregnancy and fundoscopy should be part of the pre-pregnancy screen as should assessment of renal function. Renal failure may also worsen considerably during pregnancy and such women should be managed jointly by obstetrician, renal physician, and diabetologist from pre-pregnancy onwards.

Pregnancy

As soon as pregnancy is suspected, assume that the patient is pregnant. Encourage patients to report to their GP or diabetes team if a period is a week late (individual discussion is required for those with irregular periods). As some pregnancy tests are insufficiently sensitive to diagnose pregnancy on urine testing, send a blood sample for human chorionic gonadotrophin analysis, or treat the patient as if pregnant and perform pregnancy tests on early morning urine samples at weekly intervals unless menstruation occurs. Often the patient has made the diagnosis herself using highly sensitive over-the-counter tests. Pregnant diabetic women should be referred that day by telephone to the diabetologist and obstetrician who provide joint care (most diabetologists will be happy to contact the obstetric services themselves).

In the joint diabetic/obstetric clinic, the pregnant woman is fully assessed clinically, including blood pressure measurement and renal function, and has a formal ophthalmological review. Meter-read finger-prick blood glucose testing, before each meal, after the largest meal, and occasionally during the night, is instituted if not already in progress. Her insulin is adjusted to achieve blood glucose concentrations of 4.0–5.0 mmol/l fasting and 4.0–7.0 mmol/l random. She should go to bed with a blood glucose of at least 6.0 mmol/l to reduce the risk of hypoglycaemia. The couple should be given a supply of glucagon and her partner should be taught how to use it. Hypoglycaemia is common as patients strive for normoglycaemia and patients and their partners must be warned of this. The patient should always carry glucose on her person and needs to be particularly careful to avoid hypoglycaemia if she is already caring for small children. The required insulin dose rises during pregnancy and may have doubled by term. During labour and delivery, insulin and glucose need to be infused intravenously according to a sliding scale. Within hours of delivery the insulin requirements will have dropped to the pre-pregnant dose.

A dietitian and diabetes specialist nurse or midwife trained in diabetes care should see the patient. The diabetes specialist nurse or midwife can also see her at home.

If the GP is sharing diabetes and/or obstetric care with the hospital, careful notes in the patient-held co-operation record are essential. Telephone the team if any problems are suspected.

Obstetric care will include frequent checks; for example, fortnightly for the first two trimesters and weekly in the last, and serial ultrasound scans, including examination for anomalies. Many obstetricians deliver diabetic women at 38 weeks and may have a low threshold for Caesarian section. Caesarian section should be covered by prophylactic antibiotics as there is high risk of infection.

In a diabetic pregnancy, the risks to the patient and fetus include pregnancy-induced hypertension, polyhydramnios, ketoacidosis, fetal malformation, poor fetal growth, macrosomia, sudden intrauterine death, respiratory distress syndrome, and post-partum hypoglycaemia (for both). These complications can be reduced by intensive diabetes and obstetric management but some women who have been normoglycaemic throughout pregnancy still have macrosomic babies.

One of the difficulties with care of the pregnant diabetic woman is that there is no consensus about the precise blood glucose levels to aim for, the process of obstetric care, or the type or timing of delivery. The most important factor appears to be frequent care by a team experienced in the management of diabetes in pregnancy, with close attention to detail, and 24-hour availability of immediate help (by telephone or in person) if problems arise.

Gestational diabetes

Diabetes may arise during pregnancy and is especially likely in the third trimester. Diagnostic criteria vary—many physicians use the Diabetes UK values (p. 7). Others use more stringent criteria, diagnosing diabetes if the fasting glucose is over 5.0 mmol/l or a random, postprandial value is over 7.0 mmol/l. Once diagnosed, women with gestational diabetes are treated like any other pregnant diabetic woman. After delivery, glucose tolerance may revert to normal, or remain impaired. Up to 60 per cent of women with gestational diabetes may eventually develop permanent diabetes. This is especially likely in Asian women. The maintenance of a diabetic diet and regular exercise (see p. 41) may delay or prevent the reappearance of diabetes. There is a high likelihood of gestational diabetes in further pregnancies.

Breast-feeding

Diabetic women can breast-feed. They may need to eat more carbohydrate (about 100 g or ten portions a day in those who measure this) and reduce their insulin dose according to blood glucose levels. They should snack before feeding and drink more fluid. With disturbed nights and erratic exercise patterns there is a risk of hypoglycaemia. I usually suggest that glycaemic balance is relaxed from the pregnancy normoglycaemia to around 6–9 mmol/l during this time. Do not forget that contraception needs to be restarted unless further pregnancies are planned.

Motherhood

Women sometimes forget about themselves as they rush around, cooking, cleaning, picking Johnny up from nursery school, delivering Suzanne to ballet, and more. It is even harder work if the woman has an additional paid job. The diabetes can be the last item on the agenda and the aim may be seen as 'keeping a little sugary to avoid hypoglycaemia and not testing too much because I'm busy.' The diet may be erratic, including remnants from the children's plates. Of course, they know what they ought to be doing but this is just until the children are older. A family of two can occupy a woman for 18–20 years—long enough to develop all the complications of diabetes. Mothers should be encouraged to give themselves some time for daily body maintenance—perhaps at a time when their partner is at home and can look after the children. The GP and practice nurse can keep a gentle watch on the way in which the patient is coping with her diabetes when she attends with her children, as well as ensuring that mother attends for her own check-ups.

Menopause

Blood glucose balance occasionally becomes erratic during the menopause although afterwards the insulin requirement may fall. This may not apply if the woman is given hormone replacement therapy. There are several views on this, but providing the treatment is given in truly 'replacement' doses, i.e. physiological rather than pharmacological, it seems sensible to apply the same criteria for initiating hormone replacement therapy as in non-diabetic women.

Men

Fatherhood

The diabetic father is under many of the same pressures as the diabetic mother: he may be the one looking after the children. In many cases, he may be the breadwinner. They may worry that their diabetes is going to stop them working and make them let their family down. As with working women, they may be working so hard, that they neglect themselves and their diabetes. They may ignore check-ups because they do not wish to take time off work. It may be difficult to contact them but they may be prepared to attend an evening or Saturday clinic. Being self-employed can be particularly stressful.

Libido and infections

Untreated diabetes or hyperglycaemia can reduce libido temporarily. Diabetic men may also develop candidal infection: balanitis. Both the man and his partner should be treated with antifungals. As in women, the critical factor is returning the blood glucose toward normal. Fertility is not impaired and there appears to be no problem for the fetus if the father has hyperglycaemia at conception.

Erectile dysfunction (ED)

Approximately one in three men with diabetes may experience ED, either temporarily or permanently. ED may be under-reported as the ambience of many diabetic clinics or busy surgeries is not always conducive to such sensitive discussions. Bearing in mind that it may have taken considerable courage on the patient's part to reveal this symptom, any mention of sexual difficulties should be followed up, if necessary at another appointment with appropriate privacy and time, and preferably with his partner.

The first step is to define the patient's problem. ED is the inability to develop and maintain a penile erection sufficient for sexual performance. Although some men with diabetes do have permanent ED associated with diabetic tissue damage, many have reversible ED. Reversible factors, or those suggesting another condition requiring investigation and treatment should be sought, but a final decision that the ED is due to diabetes does not mean that the patient and his partner cannot be helped.

Causes of erectile dysfunction in diabetic men

- Psychological, including anxiety and depression
- Drugs, including antihypertensives, H_2 blockers, psychotropics
- Alcohol
- Neuropathy (peripheral and/or autonomic)
- Vascular disease
- Endocrine—hypogonadism

All patients will have some psychological problems either causing or due to the ED. Some districts have psychologists trained in assessment and treatment of psychosexual problems. ED due to psychological factors may start suddenly, be associated with reduced libido, and be patchy, i.e. present with one woman and not with another, or present during masturbation but not when intercourse is attempted. Drug-related ED is common and remediable; drugs implicated include methyl dopa, reserpine, beta blockers, phenothiazines, cimetidine. Endocrine causes can be suspected by finding other evidence of hypogonadism clinically. Measure testosterone, LH, FSH, and prolactin.

Evidence of diabetic tissue damage elsewhere such as retinopathy, nephropathy, neuropathy, and peripheral vascular disease, make it more likely that the ED will be related to diabetic tissue damage. It is always worth improving blood glucose control as hyperglycaemia can cause non-specific malaise which may be associated with ED (there are obviously many other reasons for improving blood glucose balance). An erectile response to alprostadil injection demonstrates adequate vascular supply. In unresponsive patients angiography may identify treatable vascular disease. If autonomic neuropathy is evident elsewhere (e.g. with postural hypotension or problems with bladder emptying) the ED is likely to be neurogenic.

More detailed studies can be undertaken in specialist centres.

Treatment of erectile dysfunction

Do a full clinical assessment and relevant blood tests in everyone. Provide psychological support as needed. Some patients will need specialist psychosexual counselling.

Sildenafil (Viagra) is licensed for use in diabetic men with ED and may be effective in over 50 per cent of cases—depending on the severity of any vascular or neurological tissue damage. Do not prescribe sildenafil for men in whom sexual activity could be harmful (e.g. patients with unstable angina). Avoid sildenafil in patients with renal failure (creatinine clearance below 30 ml/min), hepatic failure, blood pressure below 90/50, recent history of stroke or myocardial infarction, known hereditary retinal degeneration, and in those on nitrates of any sort. Avoid it in patients with anatomical abnormalities of the penis. Sildenafil's action may be enhanced with cimetidine, ketoconazole, and erythromycin.

Start with a 50 mg dose (25 mg in the elderly or those with renal impairment) and titrate the dose as required. Patients should understand that the drug is only effective with sexual stimulation. Sildenafil may cause headache, flushing, dizziness, dyspepsia, nasal congestion, and visual changes.

Other treatments are less often used nowadays. Alprostadil can be injected intracavernosally or inserted intraurethrally. Vacuum devices can be used for men with severe neurological or vascular problems. If sildenafil is unsuccessful, refer the patient to specialist care. Do not use testosterone or androgen analogues—they are only of help if the patient has proven testosterone deficiency.

Summary

- Diabetes in one person affects the whole family.
- There is a major inherited component in the development of both Type 1 and Type 2 diabetes.

- Menstruation and the menopause can cause glycaemic imbalance.
- Diabetic women are fertile and should use contraception until pregnancy is desired.
- Pregnancy should be planned.
- A woman should try to conceive only when her blood glucose is normal. It should remain normal throughout pregnancy.
- Pregnancy in a diabetic woman requires specialist supervision to reduce the likelihood of complications to mother and fetus.
- Diabetic parents should look after themselves as well as their families.
- Diabetic men may develop erectile dysfunction. It is not always due to the diabetes and may often be reversible.

Chapter 17

Older people with diabetes

Mention diabetes and the public think of a child injecting insulin. But diabetes is predominantly a disease of the elderly. One in ten of the over-70s have diabetes. The combination of old age, diabetes, and diabetes tissue damage can require complex care from many agencies. The potential role of preventive care is considerable but its delivery can be difficult. Patient education is as important in the elderly as in the young, but it may take longer and health care professionals may not have enough time. It is well worth making time.

The onset of diabetes is rarely dramatic. Insidious ill health may be the only clue. It is therefore important to test for glycosuria in every unwell old person. However, the renal threshold often rises with age, so blood tests are better. Polyuria and nocturia may lead to incontinence or bed-wetting and the patient may reduce fluids at night to attempt to avoid this. The symptoms of prostatism may become apparent or worsen. Older patients often present with the consequences of diabetes such as infection, cardiovascular disease, or foot problems.

Management

Diet

This is as important as in younger patients but should not be introduced abruptly. The patient has had 70 years on their previous diet so is unlikely to want to change. One danger is of starvation because of overstrict interpretation of sucrose reduction or vague memories of the old low carbohydrate diet. Sudden introduction of fibre can cause abdominal discomfort. Regular meals of sufficient calorie content but not too much sugar are the most important advice for thin elderly people. For overweight patients a practical weight-reducing diet with less fat and sugar is needed.

Oral hypoglycaemic drugs

Whatever drug is used it can cause problems in the elderly. Metformin is increasingly used as it does not cause hypoglycaemia unless taken in overdose. However, its gastrointestinal side-effects and the risk of lactic acidosis in patients prone to hypoxia or with renal failure may limit its use in some people. Sulphonylureas should be used with care. They can all cause hypoglycaemia (see p. 67) and glibenclamide seems especially likely to do so. Opinions are divided between using longer-acting agents for ease of administration, or short-acting drugs to reduce the duration of hypoglycaemia if it occurs. It obviously depends on the patient. One option is gliclazide 30 M/R.

If the patient has an erratic eating pattern tolbutamide or glipizide taken with meals may be safer. Experience of repaglinide in those over 75 years old is limited.

If the target blood glucose (see p. 65) is not maintained on oral agents, insulin should be started. A single injection of long-acting insulin in the morning in addition to continued oral agents sometimes controls the glucose.

Insulin

Administering insulin causes much worry in the elderly. Many people are completely capable of giving their own insulin and adjusting the dose according to blood glucose concentration. Others, for example, people with dementia, are unable to manage any aspect of their injections. Some patients can work out what to do but because of physical disability such as visual impairment or arthritis cannot draw up or inject their insulin.

If no carer is available in the house or nearby the district nurse has to come in to give the insulin. Once-daily insulin is more practical but rarely gives good control. A single dose of very long-acting insulin such as Ultratard mixed with fast-acting insulin such as Actrapid can be used. Sometimes the district nurse can draw up sufficient insulin-filled syringes for several days' supply to be kept in the fridge. These should contain only insulins which are stable when mixed (so this is not appropriate for Ultratard and Actrapid). Pre-mixed insulins can be useful. Insulin pens may allow the patient to inject their own insulin, as may magnifiers for the syringe and drawing-up guides. In thin people care must be taken not to inject the insulin intramuscularly. Problems of timing may arise if a district nurse cannot arrive before normal breakfast time and patients occasionally have their insulin after breakfast.

If an insulin-treated patient has a very variable eating pattern, or refuses food, it can be extremely difficult to control their blood glucose. Carers can be given an insulin pen and a simple sliding scale and inject the insulin, such as lispro or aspart, after food has been eaten. A single small dose of longer-acting insulin can be given in the morning if needed.

Exercise

This is as important as in younger people and can take the form of walking or gardening as well as other activities. It is important to make the effort to keep the patient moving even if their joints are stiff and they are reluctant to leave their chair by the fire. A visit to the physiotherapist can help carers to implement simple and appropriate exercise programmes.

Blood glucose concentrations

Older people with diabetes are as much at risk of tissue damage as younger people—or more so. The same risk-reduction strategies apply, if safe and practical. As a 70-year-old may live another 20 or 30 years it is important that attention is paid to preventive care. Treatment of hypertension in the elderly reduces the risk of stroke. However, efforts to achieve normoglycaemia can put the patient at risk of hypoglycaemia which can be very dangerous in the elderly, especially if they live alone.

Donald was over 70 and lived alone. One day he was found on the floor by his neighbour. On the stove were two red-hot saucepans, burnt dry. He had clearly been preparing his lunch. His insulin kit was on the kitchen shelf. He was admitted and his profound hypoglycaemia was treated but he died some days later.

It may be safer to aim for blood glucose levels just below 10 mmol/l in frail older people allowing the occasional 11 or 13. However, polyuria should be avoided. Consider whether other medication is making matters worse—thiazides or steroids, for example. Polypharmacy can increase confusion and reduce compliance.

Hypoglycaemia

This may not be recognized and some elderly people have great difficulty understanding the concept. Although many elderly people recognize the classic symptoms (see p. 97), the symptoms may be very vague. They include malaise, confusion, forgetfulness, inactivity, sleepiness, inattention, being difficult to manage, irritability, paranoid behaviour, or coma. Carers should have a high index of suspicion. If in doubt give glucose.

Tissue damage

No new symptom should be attributed to 'just old age'. Tissue damage is common in the elderly, partly due to probable long duration of diabetes before diagnosis, and in patients who have already had 40 or 50 years of diabetes. Tissue damage should be sought at diagnosis.

Visual symptoms should always be investigated. Cataract extraction can give a new lease of life. Laser treatment should be given if required (see p. 129).

The management of **cardiac failure** may be a balancing act between resolution of cardiac symptoms and biochemical derangement. Have a high index of suspicion for cardiac ischaemia which may be doubly difficult to detect in a diabetic elderly person.

Nephropathy may develop insidiously and the first sign may be hypoglycaemia. Diuretics, recurrent urinary tract infection, non-steroidal anti-inflammatories, dehydration, and hypertension may worsen the situation.

Mobility may be affected by diabetes in many ways—reduced by stroke, foot problems, vascular disease, or neuropathy; or by osteoarthritis; and limited by poor vision or the breathlessness of cardiac disease.

Pressure sores are sadly common in the chair-bound or bed-bound diabetic patient and can rapidly turn into large holes draining foul pus. Major steps must be taken to prevent them developing by obtaining appropriate chair padding or mattresses, and by teaching relatives or carers about pressure care. Incontinence due to hyperglycaemia can hasten the process.

Foot care is vital. Many of the patients who come to amputation are elderly. All people with diabetes over the age of 60 years should have regular chiropody (at their home if necessary). Everyone caring for them should be taught about the risk of foot problems and how to prevent them. It is good practice for all health care professionals to look at the patient's feet on every visit.

Remember that autonomic neuropathy can cause **postural hypotension** and may precipitate falls. Hypotensive drugs can worsen this, so in someone with diabetes, monitoring of blood pressure treatment should include lying and standing values.

Bladder and bowel problems can be due to autonomic neuropathy or other factors. Incontinence may be precipitated by urinary tract infection. Thrush may cause severe perineal soreness which the patient is too shy to mention. Urinary retention is less common but diabetic neuropathy may add to the effects of prostatism. Constipation can be stubborn despite a high-fibre diet and may require laxatives or enemata.

Mental effects

Cerebral atherosclerosis is more frequent in people with diabetes than in the general population. Patients may have one obvious stroke but multi-infarct dementia may be commoner than is generally recognized. Occasionally, prolonged, frequent hypoglycaemia can cause confusion or memory defects, or a state of paranoia which can be very hard to manage.

Elderly people may think more slowly than youngsters and can be completely overwhelmed by the torrent of information pouring over them at diagnosis of diabetes. This can cause confusion and distress and produces much anxiety. Such patients need step-wise education, away from the bustle of a big clinic, and preferably in their own home. Treatment can often be started gently to avoid early side-effects. It is usually wise to include a close relative in the discussions with the patient's permission.

Drugs in the elderly

Diuretics Diuretic therapy can cause a raised urea and may add to the effects of early nephropathy. Diuretics can also cause hyponatraemia (worse in those on chlorpropamide) and hypokalaemia. Thiazide-induced impairment of glucose tolerance, although minor in many patients, may be sufficient to cause failure of maximal oral therapy to control the blood glucose and an alternative diuretic or antihypertensive should be found. Loop diuretics can also impair glucose tolerance.

Beta blockers Loss of warning of hypoglycaemia can be a disaster at any age, but especially in the elderly. Beta blockers can worsen the symptoms of peripheral vascular disease and may cause heart failure.

Vasodilators Drugs such as nitrates and calcium channel blockers can exacerbate postural hypotension, as can ganglion blockers, although these are less often used. The ankle swelling induced by nifedipine can be uncomfortable.

Non-steroidal anti-inflammatory drugs These are one of the most commonly prescribed drugs in the elderly. They interact with sulphonylureas to cause hypoglycaemia. However, it has been suggested that aspirin may slow the development of retinopathy. It certainly reduces the likelihood of stroke in patients with transient ischaemic attacks. Aspirin also reduces mortality after coronary thrombosis. It can reduce the blood glucose but this is rarely clinically relevant. Non-steroidal anti-inflammatory drugs should not be used in patients with nephropathy.

Carers

Often diabetes care in an elderly person is provided by a relative or professional carer. It is therefore essential that they accompany the patient to the clinic or surgery. Diabetes education should be directed to both the patient and the carer. The combination of diabetes and old age can place considerable burdens on carers and their health and well-being must be considered too. Ensure that they obtain appropriate attendance allowances if relevant. Carers must know how to manage diabetes emergencies such as hypoglycaemia or a foot infection and whom to call in an emergency.

Summary

Diabetes is a disease of the elderly.

- Tailor the treatment to the person.
- Do not strive for normoglycaemia if this is going to be dangerous.
- Diabetes tissue damage is common in elderly people.
- Choose your drugs carefully—old age and diabetes may combine to increase the likelihood of confusion with medication and cause adverse effects.
- Diabetes education is important at all ages.

Further reading

Finucane, P., and Sinclair, A. (ed) (1995). *Diabetes in old age*. John Wiley and Sons, Chichester.

Chapter 18

Diabetes in Asian and Afro-Caribbean people and other ethnic groups

People from many different ethnic backgrounds will develop diabetes. It is particularly common in the South Asian community, and also in the Afro-Caribbean community in the UK. However, every health care team will also meet diabetic patients from other backgrounds—some from well-established communities in the UK; others, refugees from recent conflicts. These include Somalia and other African nations, Afghanistan, and the Balkans.

Communication

Good communication is essential for good diabetes care. The patient must learn what diabetes is, how to care for himself, and how to stay fit. Communication can be difficult if the patient and the health care team have different ethnic and cultural backgrounds. Some barriers to communication include:

(a) staff ignorance of the patient's correct name and status;

(b) gender difference;

(c) differences in non-verbal signals;

(d) lack of a common language—the patient's incomplete or non-existent understanding of spoken and/or written English; and the doctor's inability to speak or write the patient's language;

(e) different social conventions;

(f) different dietary habits;

(g) different perceptions of health and ill-health;

(h) different understanding of the reason for seeing the health care team;

(i) different expectations of the outcome of the consultation.

Make sure that the patient understands when and where to come for their appointment. Try to reduce anxiety before and during the appointment. Arrange for an interpreter to come with the patient—preferably an independent, medically-trained interpreter. Otherwise, ask patients to bring a trusted friend or relative. Beware modification of questions or answers. Nowadays, most hospitals have access to telephone interpretation lines. Would the patient prefer to see female staff—particularly if they are going to be examined? (Many Muslim women would.) Men may prefer a male doctor.

When the patient arrives, check the pronunciation of their name and record this on the notes for future reference. Throughout the consultation make sure that the

Table 18.1 The prevalence (per cent) of diabetes (known and previously undiagnosed) in people of Afro-Caribbean, Asian, and European origin

Age (years)	Asian		Afro-Caribbean		European	
	Men	Women	Men	Women	Men	Women
20–39	2.5	1.5			0.5	0.5
40–59	12.5	9.5			3.5	6.0
60–79	25.5	20.0			6.5	8.0
40+			16.7	17.7	5.0	3.1

The male:female ratio appears to be changing. In UKPDS (see p. 29) the ratio of newly-diagnosed men:women was 3:2.
Figures from summaries in *Diabetes in the United Kingdom—1996* (British Diabetic Association)

patient understands you. Invite feedback. Ask the patient to repeat what you have said—what is wrong with him or her and how it can be put right, and, most importantly, what action he or she needs to take to get better.

Information is available in a variety of languages, for example, from Diabetes UK. Foot care leaflets written by a podiatrist, Richard Hourston, are available in nearly 30 languages from *www.diabeticfoot.org.uk.*

The treatment of diabetes is always tailored to the individual's needs. The patient must accept treatment for it to succeed. In a condition in which tissue damage develops silently until it is well-advanced, it can be hard for any patient who feels well to understand the need for careful diet, regular medication, blood-glucose testing, and regular self care and health checks. A diabetes specialist nurse or practice nurse who speaks the patient's language can be a considerable help in teaching patients about their condition.

The Asian community

How common is diabetes?

Diabetes is very common in the Asian community in Britain, occurring about four times as often as in the general population. In some communities up to one in four Asian people of working age have diabetes. The frequency increases with increasing age and older Asian patients are up to seven times as likely to have diabetes as the general population. The likelihood of diabetes appears to vary according to the place of origin and on other factors such as diet.

What kind of diabetes?

Most Asian people with diabetes, even those below the age of 30 years, have Type 2 diabetes. Type 1 diabetes is uncommon, although up to 50 per cent of patients with maturity-onset type diabetes will come to need insulin to control their blood glucose level.

Diagnosis

Diabetes may go undetected until the patient attends their doctor for another reason. It may be difficult for any patient to accept that he or she has a disease and should therefore modify his lifestyle and diet, or take medication when he or she does not feel unwell.

> A community nurse with a special interest in diabetes in Asian people spent one day a week at a day centre. Within a couple of months she had discovered previously unrecognized diabetes in 20 people.

When specifying a fasting blood test to obtain a diagnostic glucose level, ensure that the patient understands what you mean by fasting. For him or her, it may mean drinking sweet tea but not eating food, or eating in the dark but not in the light of morning. This can cause diagnostic confusion.

Diet

People of Asian origin living in Britain eat a wide variety of diets. Between a third and a half have been born in Britain and many eat a Western diet. Indeed it has been postulated that it is the unhealthy fatty and sugary Western diet which has increased the frequency of diabetes in the Asian population. It is impossible to prescribe a diet until one knows something about what a person usually eats. It is also essential to talk with the person who actually does the cooking. Ideally the dietitian should speak Asian languages and have a clear understanding of Asian diets.

The main carbohydrates in Asian diets are breads (nan, chapati, bhatura), rice, and pulses such as lentils and beans. The breads can be made with wholemeal flour, and brown rice can be used, although this may be considered inferior. Butter or ghee is often used (in some breads or to cook pilau rice) and in making curries. Much of the fat in the Asian diet is part of the cooking and the patient or the cook may not count it as such when trying to reduce dietary fat. Sugar is used in sweetmeats and festival foods, for example Mithai, Laddoo, Jalaibi, Gajer halwa, Karah parshad.

There may be strict religious rules relating to food and drink and the suspicion that a food breaches these rules may mean that the whole meal is thrown away (Table 18.2). Asian patients may prefer to have their food brought into hospital by their family. People vary in the strictness with which they observe religious rules but these must always be respected according to the patient's wishes. Vegetarians may be vegans who risk vitamin B_{12} deficiency. Other vegetarians eat dairy products. The use of ghee has religious significance and this may make it difficult to leave out of a low fat diet. Different foods may have different significance under varied circumstances. Many foods are believed to cause allergies and particular foods may be avoided in certain illnesses. Some foods are considered hot and others cold and are taken to treat certain conditions. Karela, a vegetable used in some Indian dishes, reduces the blood glucose and can cause hypoglycaemia.

Medication

Oral hypoglycaemic agents and a diabetes diet can control diabetes in many patients. Those who need insulin should be offered biosynthetic human insulin as pork-derived

Table 18.2 Dietary restrictions practised by religious and ethnic groups

HINDUS	No beef	Mostly vegetarian; fish rarely eaten; no alcohol.	Periods of fasting common.
MUSLIMS	No pork	Meat must be 'Halal'; no shellfish eaten; no alcohol.	Regular fasting, including Ramadan for 1 month.
SIKHS	No beef	Meat must be killed by 'one blow to the head'; no alcohol.	Generally less rigid eating restrictions than Hindus and Muslims.
JEWS	No pork	Meat must be kosher; only fish with scales and fins eaten.	Meat and dairy foods must not be consumed together.
RASTAFARIANS	No animal products, except milk may be consumed.	Foods must be 'I-tal' or alive, so no canned or processed foods eaten; no salt added; no coffee or alcohol.	Food should be 'organic'.

Halal meat must be bled to death and dedicated to God by a Muslim present at the killing. Kosher meat must be bled to death in the presence of a Rabbi and then be soaked and salted.

Orthodox members may adhere to all the restrictions of their religion or ethnic group. Others may adhere to only the major restrictions, especially where they are immigrant in a foreign country.

Reproduced from Table 32, *Manual of nutrition* (1985), HMSO.

or beef insulin may be against their religious beliefs. Even insulin itself may be viewed as inappropriate and stopped. This can lead to repeated admissions with severe hyperglycaemia as the patient may not wish to upset the doctor by telling him that they have not taken the treatment.

Many Asian patients will also consult an alternative practitioner. Western doctors should not take offence as alternative medicine is usual in the East and implies a 'belt and braces' approach to health care rather than lack of trust in a doctor's treatment. A variety of approaches include the advice of a hakim or vaid, Ayurvedic medicine, Hikmat, astrotherapy, urinotherapy (drinking urine is thought to help diabetes), herbal medicine, and homeopathy. Problems may arise when the alternative practitioner advises stopping the Western medicine so it does not interfere with his medicine (or vice versa), or when the alternative medicine causes toxic effects or interacts with the Western pharmaceuticals. Ask the patient what other treatment he or she is taking.

Diabetic tissue damage

Ischaemic heart disease is common in Asian people. In a series followed for 11 years in Southall, the all-cause mortality of South Asians (242/730 died) aged 30–54 at baseline was 1.5 times that of the European cohort (172/304 died). The mortality ratio for circulatory disorders was 1.8, that for heart disease 2.02. In South Asians, circulatory disorders in total accounted for 77 per cent of deaths, compared with 46 per cent in Europeans (Mather *et al.* 1998*a*). South Asian people experience greater delays in obtaining appropriate specialist help and investigation for heart disease than Europeans, even though they are more likely to seek help for chest pain (Chaturvedi *et al.* 1997). Compared with Europeans, South Asian patients are more likely to be overweight, to have a high waist: hip ratio, to have unfavourable lipid profiles, and poorer glucose control. Asian women are less likely to be physically active.

In addition to greater cardiovascular risk, recent studies show that South Asian patients are more likely to develop microalbuminuria, and they are more likely to have retinopathy and hypertension (Mather *et al.* 1998*b*). Nephropathy occurs more often and earlier in South Asian diabetic patients and they may need renal transplantation. Retinopathy and neuropathy are often severe when they are discovered, perhaps because there is a longer duration of diabetes before it is diagnosed. Foot problems do not seem as common as in other ethnic groups—possibly because they have less constricting foot wear and better personal foot care than other patients.

The Afro-Caribbean Community

Diabetes also appears to be more common in this community than in white Europeans (see Table 18.1). Afro-Caribbean patients usually have Type 2 diabetes. They are prone to be overweight and are more insulin-resistant than Europeans, but have a less unfavourable lipid profile than South Asian patients and are more physically active (Pomerleau *et al.* 1999). Perhaps because of this they have a lower rate of coronary disease than one might expect, but they are prone to resistant hypertension. Calcium channel antagonists appear particularly useful in this group, but several hypotensive agents are usually needed to improve blood pressure. Blood glucose control may also be difficult, and Afro-Caribbean patients also appear to have a greater risk of hyperosmolar, non-ketotic hyperglycaemic states.

Refugees

Increasing numbers of people from many nations are seeking asylum in the UK. They may have know diabetes or it may be diagnosed during health checks. Refugees have often fled atrocities and may have been badly injured—both physically and emotionally. They may have had minimal diabetes care in their country of origin—erratically available, impure insulin of unknown type; dilute insulin (e.g. 20 units/ml); infected injections sites; and no knowledge of diet or tissue damage. The new diagnosis of diabetes is yet another shock, as is the discovery of established tissue damage. Such patients may have little family or other support and be living in basic conditions. Their uncontrolled diabetes puts them at particular risk of infections such as tuberculosis, and injuries (gunshot, machete, torture) may not have healed properly. They may also have malaria, intestinal parasitaemia, HIV, and hepatitis B and C. Remember that diabetic patients and staff treating them will be monitoring finger-prick blood glucose and some will be injecting insulin.

Find the right interpreter, perform a full assessment, treat any associated problems, and control the diabetes. Find and use local appropriate support groups. It is very rewarding to see someone who has never had proper diabetes care change from a terrified, emaciated teenager into a smiling, well-nourished, healthy young woman fit enough to enjoy school.

Summary

+ Good communication is essential for full diabetes education and care.

+ Respect religious and cultural wishes.

+ Diabetes is very common in South Asian people, and also common in Afro-Caribbean people.

+ Reduce delays in diagnosis and appropriate treatment.

+ Screen for, and treat, risk factors and tissue damage.

+ Dietary advice must be tailored to the person's individual needs—talk to the person who prepares the food.

+ Remember you may not be the patient's only health adviser.

+ Refugees may have physical and emotional injuries and other health problems, with poor previous diabetes care.

+ Refugees may have continuing problems in obtaining proper diabetes care and appropriate standards of living.

References and further reading

British Diabetic Association (1995). *Diabetes in the United Kingdom—1996*. British Diabetic Association, 10 Queen Anne Street, London W1G 9LH.

Chaturvedi, N. *et al.* (1997). Lay diagnosis and health-care-seeking behaviour for chest pain in south Asians and Europeans. *Lancet*, **350**, 1578–83.

Greenhalgh, P.M. (1997). Diabetes in British South Asians: nature, nurture, and culture. *Diabetic Medicine*, **14**, 10–18.

Mather, H.M. *et al.* (1998*a*). Mortality and morbidity from diabetes in South Asians and Europeans: 11-year follow-up of the Southall Diabetes Survey, London, UK. *Diabetic Medicine*, **15**, 53–9.

Mather, H.M. *et al.* (1998*b*). Comparison of prevalence and risk factors for microalbuminuria in South Asians and Europeans with Type 2 diabetes mellitus. *Diabetic Medicine*, **15**, 672–7.

McAvoy, R.R. and Donaldson, L.J. (1990). *Health care for Asians*. Oxford University Press, Oxford.

Pomerleau, J. *et al.* (1999). Factors associated with obesity in South Asians, Afro-Caribbean and European women. *International Journal of Obesity and Related Metabolic Disorders*, **23**, 25–33.

Chapter 19

Work

Diabetes is not a problem in most jobs. However, when jobs are in short supply employers may pass over someone who has diabetes, which employers do not always understand, in favour of someone without a medical condition. This means that people with diabetes should ensure that they gain as many qualifications as possible and take every opportunity for further training and other ways of improving their curriculum vitae.

Fear of being passed over for a job or dismissed may lead people with diabetes into concealing their condition. If the patient is on insulin or sulphonylurea drugs, or has tissue damage which may impede their functioning, they must tell employers that they have diabetes, especially in any post in which hypoglycaemia or any disability from tissue damage could place them or others at risk. Any employee who drives in relation to his work must inform his employer of his diabetes.

Solely diet-treated diabetes is not a barrier to employment unless the person has tissue damage which impedes function relevant to the job.

Limitations on employment

Patients treated with oral hypoglycaemic drugs

Patients may find that there are differences in employment for those on metformin only, as compared with those taking sulphonylureas. There is little risk of hypoglycaemia for people taking metformin alone, and if this controls the diabetes, changing to metformin may help a patient's employment prospects. Patients with tablet-treated diabetes are not usually permitted to join the police, armed services, or fire brigade, or to pilot aircraft. People already working in the police and fire service are usually permitted to continue, although their role may be changed. Merchant seamen who develop diabetes requiring tablet treatment are usually allowed to remain at sea, subject to a regular medical check. Patients may be allowed to drive large goods vehicles, passenger-carrying vehicles, or main-line trains, if they can prove that their diabetes is well controlled and that they have no tissue damage impairing relevant functions (e.g. poor vision, numb feet).

Patients treated with insulin

There are more limitations here because of the greater risk of hypoglycaemia. People with insulin-treated diabetes are not permitted to join the armed services, police, or fire service, become professional divers, work on an offshore oil rig, become merchant seamen, drive large goods vehicles or passenger-carrying vehicles, or control trains or aeroplanes. They may also be barred from working in some high-risk areas alone (e.g. supervising an electricity generating station or substation, signalman). Jobs in which hypoglycaemia could be fatal, such as steeplejack or scaffolder, or in which a hypoglycaemic person could be injured or cause injury by machinery are also inappropriate. However, people who develop the need for insulin-treatment whilst employed in some of these areas may be allowed to stay. Several fire-fighters on insulin have regained fully-operational status in Britain recently. The patient will have to prove that he is in full control of his condition, that there is no risk of hypoglycaemia, and that he has no tissue damage that limits relevant function. Such patients (and those on tablets) should be referred to a consultant diabetologist for assessment.

Sometimes patients face the dilemma of health or work:

> Bill was a bus driver. He was treated with oral hypoglycaemics but it was apparent that these were not sufficient to control his blood glucose. He was advised to start insulin treatment. He refused because he would lose his job. Over the next two years his hyper-glycaemia increased. Diabetic retinopathy was detected. He steadfastly refused to consider insulin despite warnings that his health might be permanently damaged.

A changing situation

The situation is changing as better methods for self-monitoring became more widely available and employers become better informed about diabetes. Cases must be assessed individually, and it is prudent to advise reassessment or regular checks as diabetes is a progressive disease.

One of the problems faced by people with diabetes is the different backgrounds of occupational medical officers. Diabetes is a rapidly moving field and occupational physicians may not always be aware of the extent to which people with diabetes can now monitor and control their condition. A patient who is experiencing difficulties with gaining employment or with their employer should ensure that any medical officer appointed by the company communicates with his GP and with his consultant diabetologist.

Work record and time off

American statistics (Drury 1985) indicate that among people aged between 20 and 64 years, 17 per cent of the general population, and 50 per cent of people with diabetes considered themselves limited in some way in the kind or amount of work they could do about the house or in employment. However, these perceptions of limitation do not actually impede full-time work in most instances. Studies of sick leave and disability in people with diabetes have shown variable results. (Greenwood and Raffle 1988). An American survey (Mayfield et al. 1999) studied people aged 25 years or over. There were 1502 people with diabetes and 20 405 without. Work disability secondary to illness/disability (lasting for half of the year 1987) occurred in 25.6 per cent of those with diabetes and 7.8 per cent of those without. People with diabetes earned less than those without. A Scandinavian study (Wandell et al. 1997) compared people with diabetes with those without diabetes but either hypertension or musculoskeletal problems, and with people with no problem. People with diabetes had lower incomes and were more likely to be on a disability pension than those with hypertension or no problem. Diabetic patients had more sick days and were more likely to have psychological problems than healthy people. A few people with diabetes with recurrent admissions for glycaemic instability, or who develop major tissue damage, may have prolonged sick leave. This may enhance an employer's negative image of diabetes.

Diabetes is a registrable disability in terms of employment and this may increase employment chances in businesses keen to fill their quota of people registered disabled. However, most people with diabetes do not register.

Effects of the job upon diabetes

Sedentary work

This poses few problems. However, if the person is more active at home at weekends, they may need a different dose of tablets or insulin for weekdays and weekends. If someone is normoglycaemic during a sedentary working day, unexpected exercise needs to be covered by extra carbohydrate. A change from an active job to a sedentary one may need a reduction in food eaten and/or a reduction in hypoglycaemic treatment. Patients may need to guard against weight gain.

Physical work

The person needs to eat enough to fuel the work. This is not usually a problem, but some people with newly-diagnosed diabetes are frightened of eating the wrong foods and reduce their diet. Insulin-treated patients, and many on sulphonylureas need regular snacks. People working on building sites and in similar industries must wear protective footwear.

Shift work

This can prove difficult for patients on insulin, and sometimes for those on sulphonylureas. They need to balance the timing of food intake, exertion, and insulin. One regimen is to have evenly spaced meals and snacks when awake, including one before going to sleep. An injection of medium-acting insulin is given before sleeping, and short-or very short-acting insulin is given before meals with an insulin pen. Encourage patients to discuss their work pattern with their doctor—many do not do so and find it difficult to resolve their glucose balance.

Work involving travelling

Driving is discussed on pp. 185–8. The person must not become hypoglycaemic while driving. If long journeys are involved, insulin-treated patients should snack and test blood glucose at least every two hours. If possible the patient should take packed meals as it may be hard to find the components of a diabetes diet on the road. In any case, anyone who travels frequently or for long distances should carry sufficient carbohydrate for an emergency full meal in the car.

The businessman or woman

Some of the hazards of the traditional business life are smoking, alcohol, and rich food. As smoking in the work place becomes less acceptable, patients should hopefully find it easier to give up, and to ask that meetings are smoke free. People with diabetes can drink in moderation (21 units a week for men and 14 units a week for women) but must never drink on an empty stomach. To reduce intake alcohol can be alternated with non-alcoholic drinks or diluted. Eating out may place a strain on the diabetes diet but most restaurants will grill meat or fish and provide plain potatoes, rice, or pasta, with bread to top up. Salad or vegetables and fruit are usually available and there is no need to have butter, dressing, sugar, or cream.

Colleagues at work

People with diabetes on sulphonylureas or insulin should tell their work colleagues that they have diabetes. For insulin-treated patients it is sensible to teach one or two colleagues what to do in the event of hypoglycaemia. Everyone on insulin should carry glucose and a supply at work is essential. Some patients keep a supply of insulin and blood testing kit at work—this must be locked away. People who give insulin injections at work should do so openly in a clean environment with explanations to avoid stigmatization as a drug abuser. The same applies to finger-prick blood glucose testing. Many people do not test at work at all and miss valuable information this way.

Diabetic tissue damage

This may be present when a person applies for a job, or may develop during employment. People with diabetes may fail to appreciate the existence or significance of complications. Visual loss from diabetic eye disease, retinopathy, or cataracts, can obviously affect someone's job. Cataracts should be extracted promptly. Retinopathy or its treatment can cause visual loss—new vessels may cause vitreous haemorrhage, maculopathy can cause severe visual loss, laser photocoagulation can reduce peripheral vision. Peripheral vascular disease may limit walking distance, cardiac disease may limit exertion. Nephropathy may require time-consuming treatment. Autonomic neuropathy may be embarrassing (for example gustatory sweating or diabetic diarrhoea) or dangerous (for example postural hypotension which may limit where the person may work with safety). Neuropathy in the hands may limit jobs requiring fine finger work, and in the feet may cause problems for those relying on foot work. Diabetic foot problems may cause months off work and may be repeatedly exacerbated if, for example, the job involves standing all day. Amputation or the need for crutches or a wheelchair may limit where a patient can work and what he can do. Fears about work may delay a patient seeking or accepting treatment for foot disease and other complications.

> Andrew had major diabetic tissue damage, including peripheral neuropathy and had already had one below knee amputation due to osteomyelitis. His artificial leg rubbed but

he ignored the ulcer which appeared on the stump and continued to walk on it. He developed osteomyelitis in the stump. He required prolonged admission. Despite repeated advice he went back to work on his artificial leg because his company were unhappy about his ability to escape on crutches or a wheelchair if there was a fire. Further ulceration appeared in the stump and he needed weeks off work. He became very depressed.

Retirement, superannuation, and pensions

People who develop diabetes after enrolling in a pension scheme are unlikely to face problems. However, some pension schemes may refuse to accept people with diabetes in which case the person can make personal arrangements. This problem may prevent a person with diabetes being employed. Insurance companies (for example those linked with pension or superannuation schemes) vary enormously in their approach to people with diabetes. Insurance companies and financial risk assessors have to rely on old data to assess the effects of diabetes upon morbidity and mortality. As diabetes care has changed greatly in the last ten years, it is hoped that morbidity and mortality may be reduced. The degree to which this may be so is clearly difficult to predict. These factors and the different depths of knowledge of insurance companies and others means that there is considerable variability in insurance companies' attitudes to people with diabetes. Some companies refuse to provide any form of life insurance, especially if the person has tissue damage, and others demand varying increases in premium. The forms requesting information suggest that some companies have failed to appreciate current standards of treatment and self-monitoring; for example, some still assume that all patients rely on urine glucose testing. The size and type of firm employing the patient may also influence the outcome, as will the patient's salary and hence anticipated pension. Some patients opt for early retirement, for social reasons or because of their diabetes. They need to be very careful that this will not cause a major financial shortfall. Remind patients that their GP and diabetes consultant can help by providing accurate up-to-date information in their support if problems arise. They should also be aware that it is in their interests to shop around for insurance and pension schemes if the opportunity arises. Diabetes UK will provide up-to-date advice.

Summary

- Diabetes rarely impedes the opportunity or capacity for employment.
- Ignorance on the part of employers and insurers may reduce a diabetic person's chances in the employment market.
- Factors which do influence employability are the risk of hypoglycaemia and its consequences, and tissue damage which may reduce function.
- People with diabetes need good qualifications and should be able to demonstrate that they can control their diabetes well.
- The GP and diabetologist can support a patient by educating employers.

References

Drury, T.F. (1985). Disability among adult diabetics. In *Diabetes in America*, pp. XXVIII–1–22. National Diabetes Data Group, National Institutes of Health 85–1468.

Greenwood, R.H., and Raffle, P.A.B. (1988). Diabetes Mellitus. In *Fitness for work* (ed F.C. Edwards, and R.I. McCallum), pp. 233–44. Oxford University Press.

Mayfield, J.A., *et al.* (1999). Work disability and diabetes. *Diabetes care*, 22, 1105–9.

Wandell, P.E., *et al.* (1997). Psychic and socioeconomic consequence with diabetes compared to other chronic conditions. *Scandinavian Journal of Social Medicine*, 25, 39–43.

Essential reading

Diabetes employment handbook (1992). British Diabetic Association (BDA).
A guide to finding and keeping work if you have diabetes. BDA.
Employing people who have diabetes. BDA.

Chapter 20

Travel

This section considers modes of travel and then some factors relating to journeys in this country and abroad.

Walking

For many, walking to work or to the shops is part of daily routine. Brisk walking on a regular basis may reduce cardiovascular risk and should be encouraged. It may be a more acceptable form of exercise to many people than jogging or training in a gym. People on insulin or glucose-lowering tablets should ensure that they carry glucose on their person. For long walks or if walking at a time when they would normally be sedentary, or just before a meal they may need to eat a snack.

Expeditions on foot, especially when carrying a rucksack, require huge amounts of carbohydrate to fuel them, especially if the person is taking insulin. The insulin dose covering the period of the expedition and twelve hours afterwards should be reduced by 20 to 50 per cent. The person will need three large meals each day, and it is sensible to eat hourly in between. On very strenuous expeditions involving much uphill work or very heavy loads, the person should eat two double snacks (i.e. containing twice the normal amount of carbohydrate of a usual snack) between each meal and between the evening meal and bed. Sufficient extra food should be carried to ensure that the person could safely spend the night away from base in an emergency.

Cycling

This is part of everyday life for many people and helps to keep them fit. For those at risk of hypoglycaemia there is the danger of a road traffic accident. The cyclist should wear a helmet and eat sufficient to avoid hypoglycaemia. The danger time is cycling home from work, or the end of a long journey. On a long journey or mountain bicycling, insulin should be reduced and carbohydrate intake increased as described for a long walk. Some of the carbohydrate can be taken as liquid.

Driving

Form D100 (January 1991) from the Driver and Vehicle Licensing Agency, 'What you need to know about driver licensing,' states:

> If after your licence has been granted, you develop a medical condition or your medical condition worsens, you **must** inform the Licensing Centre **at once** . . . You must declare any medical condition which is likely to last more than 3 months and may affect your ability to drive . . .

It is essential that you report the following:

> Epilepsy . . . sudden attacks of disabling giddiness or fainting . . . heart pain (angina) while driving, any heart condition causing loss of consciousness, loss of awareness or visual blurring, diseases of the nervous system including strokes, TIAs, . . . visual problems affecting both eyes such as cataracts, glaucoma or laser treatment, disabilities of limbs or spine, diabetes treated by insulin or tablets.

The DVLA are quite clear that people applying for a licence or with an existing one must follow these rules and this is enforceable by law. Diabetic patients on diet alone do not need to notify the DVLA unless they have notifiable complications. Tablet-treated patients will usually be allowed to keep their 'till 70' licence. Diabetic drivers on insulin will be usually be given a three-year licence renewable on re-application. It is the patient's obligation to inform the DVLA—a surprising number of patients do not. An equally surprising number continue to drive with some of the problems listed above.

> Mary, a middle-aged woman on insulin treatment, applied for renewal of her driving licence. Her physician was unaware that she was driving at all until a form arrived from the DVLA. In answer to the statutory questions the physician had to reply that Mary had severe hypoglycaemic episodes without warning, bilateral proliferative retinopathy for which there had been extensive laser treatment, a myocardial infarct followed by angina, and a stroke with hemiparesis.

The visual requirement is 'reading a number plate with the standard size letters and figures 79.4 mm high in good daylight at a distance of 20.5 m (about 23 paces).' This is approximately between 6/9 and 6/12 on the Snellen chart. However, field loss and the dispersal of bright light by cataracts (limiting night driving) will also be considered. A point which is not made by the DVLA but which precludes driving with pedals, is severe peripheral neuropathy—by the time someone with numb feet and poor position sense has found the brake it may be too late. An automatic car may well be safer for people with any degree of neuropathy, but it is still necessary to be able to feel the pedals.

Motor insurance companies regard diabetes as a material fact about which they should be informed immediately it is diagnosed. They would also regard the development of any of the conditions listed above as material facts. Furthermore, insurance companies might not cover a patient who had failed to inform the DVLA of their diabetes.

> Dennis had had diabetes for over twenty years. He was insulin-treated. He lost awareness of hypoglycaemia around the time that he developed renal impairment. He was admitted with severe hypoglycaemia, having been involved in a major road traffic accident. The accompanying police had already discovered that Dennis had not notified the DVLA about his diabetes. He was fined for that and also charged with driving while under the influence of a drug (insulin).

Insurance companies vary widely in their premiums to drivers with diabetes—one study showed that one company quoted double the premium of another for the same case. Drivers should obtain several quotations or use a broker. Diabetes UK can be of help.

Warnings to drivers

This section highlights some of the advice above.

Diet-treated patients Should be warned to contact the DVLA if they are started on oral hypoglycaemic drugs or insulin.

Starting insulin or changing the regimen These patients should be warned not to drive for a week (or more depending on individual problems) after starting insulin treatment or changing the treatment, for example from one type of insulin to another or from once a day to twice a day.

Loss or reduction of warning symptoms of hypoglycaemia Such patients should be warned not to drive. Some may be able to do so if they eat and measure their blood glucose every time they get into the car; and they eat and measure glucose hourly during a journey.

Eye problems Diabetic drivers who develop cataracts, exudative retinopathy, maculopathy, proliferative retinopathy, or who have had laser treatment, should drive only after assessment by an ophthalmologist. These drivers must inform the DVLA of their condition. (If in doubt about other eye problems consult an ophthalmologist.)

Leg or foot problems These patients should be individually assessed for safety to drive. They should inform the DVLA of any problem that is unlikely to resolve in 3 months which might impede their finding or using the pedals normally; they should also avoid driving while it is being treated. Patients with foot ulcers do not always realize that their insurance companies would regard this a material fact. Neuropaths may not realize that they have neuropathy, so their doctor must tell them. Both lack of sensation and muscle weakness may preclude driving.

What should a patient do if hypoglycaemic behind the wheel?

STOP! Hypoglycaemia may produce a compulsion to drive on. The patient should pull in and stop the instant it is safe to do so, turn off the ignition, and remove the keys. He must eat glucose and move out of the driving seat if possible, preferably by sliding over into the passenger seat. Diabetes UK advises patients to get out of the car if safe, so that they are no longer in charge of the vehicle. However, this may be extremely dangerous in the midst of a busy road or on a motorway as hypoglycaemic people often have no concept of danger and may be confused and unsteady on their feet.

After taking glucose the person should eat a carbohydrate snack and be absolutely certain that he has fully recovered and that there is no further risk of hypoglycaemia before driving off. This means waiting at least half an hour, or more.

Vocational driving

People with insulin-treated diabetes may not apply for large goods vehicle or passenger carrying vehicle licences. People with existing LGV (large good vehicle) or PCV (passenger-carrying vehicle) licences who start insulin therapy must stop driving and inform the DVLA. In some instances this also applies to sulphonylurea-treated patients, although people with tablet-treated diabetes may apply for LGV or PCV licences. If they subsequently need insulin they may lose their job. Local authorities and the Metropolitan police (responsible for licensing taxi drivers), and employers of drivers of emergency vehicles (such as fire, ambulance, police) may apply additional, more stringent criteria than the DVLA in some cases.

People with diabetes on insulin who have ordinary car licences can apply for C1 licences (vehicles weighing 3.5–7.5 tonnes) and D1 licences (mini buses) if they satisfy stringent diabetes safety criteria (contact Diabetes UK for advice).

Travel at home and abroad

People with diabetes can travel wherever they wish. However, it is prudent to plan the journey and to ensure that their diabetes and their bodies are in a fit state to travel; that they are well supplied with diabetes management drugs and equipment; and that they have considered what to do if things go wrong. Diabetes UK issues a series of travel guides for most parts of the world. Clearly, the degree of preparation depends on where the patient is going, for how long, and how remote or potentially hazardous it is.

Check the diabetes and the body

Is the diabetes stable?

Check blood glucose balance. People with very erratic blood glucose balance should resolve the problem before travelling. Travelling with recurrent, severe hypoglycaemia is ill-advised.

Is there evidence of tissue damage?

Anyone with diabetic foot problems should see a chiropodist before travelling. Holidays are a common cause of diabetes foot ulcers—new shoes, no socks, long, hot walks, sand and grit, may easily result in neglected minor injury, ulcer, infection, gangrene, amputation—a sadly frequent sequence. People with untreated retinal neovascularization should not travel (unless essential) until it has been treated and is resolving. Flying would appear to be particularly unwise because of pressure changes. Other tissue damage such as cardiac, renal, or peripheral vascular disease, may require special consideration or further treatment.

Have they adequate diabetes supplies and to spare?

Encourage your patients to give you plenty of notice so that there is time to obtain prescriptions. They need to take twice as much (in very remote areas, three times) of all their diabetes supplies as they need. Ask if the patient has enough:

Insulin (bottles, disposable pens, or cartridges)

Tablets—diabetic and others

Syringes and needles or pen (take a spare) and pen needles

Needle clipper (B-D Safeclip)

Blood glucose measuring strips and meter if used

Finger-pricking equipment—lancets and platforms

Emergency glucose (for example Dextrosol or Hypostop)

Glucagon (with syringe and needle)

Do they need immunization or prophylactic treatment?

People with diabetes should have all the relevant immunizations and their tetanus immunization should always be up-to-date. These may temporarily upset blood glucose balance. Patients must also take antimalarials if appropriate. Advice about food and water hygiene is essential—gastroenteritis abroad can be a disaster for someone with diabetes—every year several such cases arrive at our airports. Antiemetics, motion-sickness pills, and anti-diarrhoeals, with a course of antibiotics (for example, amoxycillin or erythromycin) are useful for the traveller abroad. Prescribe these if relevant.

Identification

The person with diabetes should carry a diabetes card, preferably with a message in the language(s) of the country(ies) to be visited. The message should be:

> I am a diabetic on insulin/tablets. If I am found ill please give me 2 teaspoons of sugar in a small amount of water or three of the glucose tablets which I am carrying. If I fail to recover in 10 minutes, please call an ambulance.

Translations into most languages can be obtained from Diabetes UK or the relevant embassy or tourist office. Anyone carrying syringes is likely to be stopped by security or customs, and while there is no problem if the patient can clearly identify himself as having diabetes, failure to do so immediately may lead to lengthy delays. For patients with multiple tissue damage, a doctor's letter summarizing their medical history and therapy can be very helpful if the patient is taken ill abroad.

The journey

The main aim is to avoid hypoglycaemia while travelling. It can be hard enough to find one's way around a British bus depot. Imagine trying to explain to a Tibetan policeman that you are standing by yourself in the snow because your yak has bolted and you have lost the way to your yurt. Now imagine trying to do it when hypoglycaemic.

Patients on diet alone should endeavour to adhere to the general principles of their diet and pay attention to areas affected by tissue damage if relevant. Otherwise they rarely experience problems travelling. Nor do those on metformin. Patients on oral agents rarely encounter problems but should beware of hypoglycaemia if exercise is increased or meals delayed. Some may reduce their dose of tablets slightly on the day of travel.

Some patients take a holiday from their diabetes and leave their testing kit behind. Yet it is under unfamiliar surroundings that they most need to know their blood glucose. Insulin-treated patients should test their blood glucose every 4–6 hours while travelling a long way. (More often if driving themselves, see p. 185.) They may become very confused about insulin treatment. The easiest stratagem is to consider the day of travel as being from breakfast in the country they are leaving until breakfast in their destination. During that day they should reduce the insulins which are acting while travelling, but be prepared to take a small extra dose (say 2–6 units fast-acting insulin) before an extra meal if the breakfast-breakfast time exceeds 24 hours and the blood glucose is 11 mmol/l or more. This is obviously easier if the patient is using fast-acting insulin from a pen. Patients should eat something every 2–3 hours. If planning to sleep, they should check that their glucose is over 6 mmol/l and have a snack if it is lower.

All diabetes medication and equipment should be carried personally in hand luggage, bags, or pockets, perhaps divided between the patient and a relative or companion (although the patient must carry it all through customs and security). It should never be entrusted to baggage handled by anyone else or out of sight of its owner.

Unusual foreign food

Some patients worry greatly about being able to stick to their diet in a hotel in Morecambe or on the Costa Brava. While it may be hard to find exactly the right balance of carbohydrate, fat, and protein, all countries have a staple carbohydrate—potato, bread, rice, pasta, maize, beans, etc. Obvious sugar and fat can be avoided. It is usually possible to find cooked vegetables, salad, and fruit. All uncooked fruit and salad must be washed or peeled very carefully to reduce the risk of gastroenteritis. Patients should drink only bottled water (breaking the seal themselves) or other canned, bottled, or packaged drinks with a previously unbroken seal. Alcohol, of course, is self-sterilizing but as always should be taken in moderation. A few weeks on a less than perfect diet is not the disaster some patients imagine. If they are very worried they can always carry some food with them, providing the country permits this (Australia has limits on what can be imported, for example). It is, in any case, prudent to take some food in case of delays while travelling.

Hazards abroad

Heat

Britons are not always used to heat. People with diabetes may be more likely to be sunburned on neuropathic areas, and severe burning can cause hyperglycaemia as well as the risk of infection.

> Clare, a young woman with peripheral neuropathy went to Portugal. She spent each day sunbathing by the hotel pool. She covered herself in sunscreen. One day, she paddled in the pool and returned to her sun-lounger. When she went to bed that night she found that she had scarlet 'socks'—her neuropathic feet had been burned where the water had washed the sunscreen off. Blisters developed, followed by infection and she had to come home early.

Heat can increase the rate of insulin absorption from the injection site. Increased sweating may cause dehydration and saline depletion if combined with hyperglycaemia.

Insulin deteriorates if heated. Cool bags for insulin are available from several manufacturers. Care must be taken not to freeze the insulin. It should be kept at the bottom of the hotel fridge if available.

Cold

Insulin is absorbed more slowly in the cold. It may all be released later when the person warms up. This may cause unexpected hypoglycaemia (e.g. during the *après ski* and combined with alcohol). Hypoglycaemia and cold are a potentially lethal combination (see p. 105). Patients with peripheral vascular disease should insulate their feet from the cold to avoid frostbite. Patients with cardiac disease may find that the cold weather brings on their angina.

Infection

Skin infections are common in returning diabetic travellers—they include fungal infections, e.g. athlete's foot or thrush. Infections of minor wounds, especially on the feet are frequent. Chest and urinary infection may cause hyperglycaemia which is why a short course of antibiotics can be useful. Patients must remember to increase their tablets (if this is within the safe dosage range) or their insulin dose if their blood glucose levels rise. Remind them what to do before they set off.

Medical aid abroad

150 million people in the world have diabetes. Specialist diabetes care is available in most countries, but access to it is very variable. Any patient going to a foreign country for an extended visit should be given a contact for diabetes help in that country. The International Diabetes Federation (IDF) can provide addresses for member associations and help with contacts. For Europe the organization is IDF (Europe) (see p. 220). Medical care can often be excellent but, as in any country, not every medical team is familiar with diabetes.

> A diabetic man went on holiday in South Asia. Towards the end of the holiday he developed diarrhoea and vomiting and felt very unwell. He went to a doctor who measured his blood glucose. He was told it was very high but no treatment was advised—not even an increase in his insulin dose. Because he had not been told to alter his insulin the patient did not like to do so himself. No one was ever able to establish how he spent the last few days of his holiday. He could not remember and could not even recall his flight home when he was admitted from the airport in severe diabetic ketoacidosis. The prolonged flight had exacerbated the dehydration.

Travel insurance is essential. The patient must declare his diabetes as most insurance policies have small print clauses relating to existing illness. This also applies to insurance arranged via a travel agent or transport company. The premium varies from company to company. It is important to get a policy which guarantees flight home if necessary. Even trips in Britain can become very expensive if the patient has to return home or be admitted to hospital and it is worth considering travel insurance here too.

General advice

Whether the person with diabetes is going away for a day or a year, in their home country or abroad, they must always allow for the unexpected. As I write this I have just heard that a London train was delayed tonight because there was a llama on the line.

Summary

- Walking and cycling are good exercise. Patients should ensure they have enough food to fuel it if necessary and avoid hypoglycaemia.
- Drivers with diabetes taking tablets or insulin must inform the DVLA of their condition. All people with diabetes who develop tissue damage likely to affect their ability to drive safely must also inform the DVLA.
- Drivers must inform their insurance company of their diabetes and any relevant tissue damage.
- People with diabetes who travel should prepare for the unexpected.
- Travel insurance removes the anxiety about what may happen if there is a problem.
- Planning includes a check up of their body and their diabetes, ensuring supplies of diabetes treatment and equipment, and other drugs and immunization where relevant.
- Encourage the patient to obtain the relevant Diabetes UK travel guide.
- They must carry a diabetes card in the language of their destination(s).
- Aim to avoid hypoglycaemia while travelling.
- Having diabetes should not stop a person enjoying a holiday or experimenting with foreign food.

Chapter 21

Diabetes in primary care

The primary care team know the patient, his circumstances, and his family. They can place his diabetes in perspective in relation to his total health care. General practitioners are therefore in a good position to provide diabetes care. This care is convenient as the patient usually lives nearby. However, to provide the standards of diabetes care which will keep the patient alive and well, a health care team must have specific training in diabetes care, see sufficient people to gain experience in diabetes and how it affects patients, and keep their knowledge up to date.

Each primary care team is different. A doctor will decide for himself whether he wishes to provide specialized diabetes care for his patients, and whether he has the training and resources to do so. In many instances a practical solution is to share care with a specialist diabetes team co-ordinated by a consultant diabetologist. Each general practitioner and his local diabetologist must come to an agreement about which patients or which aspects of diabetes each should care for. With our scarce resources, duplication of care should be avoided, but neither should we fail to provide an aspect of care because we think the other is doing it. This calls for good and frequent communication about diabetes care in general and about individual patients in particular. It is therefore vital to establish good and reliable channels of communication at the outset, overcoming the potential barriers of hospital switchboards and protective receptionists.

Setting up a diabetes service in primary care

How many diabetic patients are you likely to have?

A list of 3000 patients will include about 100 people with diabetes—more if a large proportion of your list are elderly or Asian people. Most of the diabetic patients on your list will have Type 2 diabetes. About 10–25 patients will have Type 1 diabetes.

Diabetes register

First find your patients. If you do not know who has diabetes you cannot treat them. A diabetes register (which can be a simple box of cards or a computer list) is a prerequisite. To start with this may rely on memory and flagging the notes as diabetic patients are seen by practice staff for any reason. Prescription records for glucose-lowering medication may help. One staff member should be responsible for maintaining an up to date diabetes register.

What resources do you have?

All surgeries have the minimum accommodation—a consulting room, somewhere for urine and blood testing, a waiting area, and record storage. However, if you are planning a diabetes service in which the practice nurse sees patients as well as the doctor, with a dietitian, or a chiropodist or with group education sessions, rooms need to be found for them too. For a clinic in which all personnel are present at the same time this can mean a lot of rooms unavailable to other patients or staff for a whole session.

Staff

The minimum staff is one doctor. However, some facets of diabetes care do not need to be carried out by a doctor, and some are better done by other health professionals (for example, dietetics, chiropodists). Many surgeries now have a practice nurse.

People with diabetes should have regular access to a dietitian and chiropodist, and benefit greatly from the help of a specialist diabetes nurse. It may be possible to share these personnel with the hospital, other practices, or the community services. If not, patients should be referred to the hospital service for dietetic, chiropody, and diabetes specialist nurse advice.

Training

Unless the doctor has had recent training in diabetes he should attend a training course. In one study 83 per cent of general practitioners expressed interest in learning more about diabetes. Training may include the national postgraduate course, which moves from centre to centre (ask Diabetes UK for the current organizer), a local course, or the Primary Care Diabetes UK course at the University of Warwick. A period as a clinical assistant in a diabetic clinic can be helpful and has the added advantage of providing experience of many patients with diabetes. All staff participating in the clinic also need training, especially the practice nurse who may feel very vulnerable if she has not worked with people who have diabetes for some time and is given responsibility for running the clinic.

Eye examination for retinopathy must be performed by staff specifically trained in the assessment of diabetic patients—through local schemes with diabetes-accredited optometrists, retinal phographic schemes, or other ophthalmologist-approved methods.

Time

Diabetes consultations are not quick. It can take 30 to 60 minutes for a doctor to assess a new diabetic patient thoroughly. Annual reviews take 20 minutes for the doctor's review and 30 minutes for the nurse's review. Add receptionist's and clerical time and the total is about one hour per patient. Visits for glucose balance usually take 10 to 20 minutes. Elderly patients and those with communication problems take longer. Education sessions may take 15 to 60 minutes and as several topics need to be covered, each patient may need several sessions. This is where group sessions are helpful, but each patient needs individual time too.

Some general practitioners see people with diabetes as part of their usual list. Others establish separate clinics for people with diabetes and one doctor sees his own and his

Equipment

Glucose testing meter (See *MIMS* for current list). The equipment must be calibrated correctly and well-maintained. Staff using it must be trained properly (the manufacturer will usually arrange this). If your local hospital runs a quality assurance scheme take part in it. Otherwise the manufacturer may be able to help with standard samples.

Sphygmomanometer A normal-sized and a large (thigh) cuff are needed.

Monofilaments For testing touch sensation. (Bailey Instruments 0161 860 5849; Smith and Nephew 01623 722337.)

Tuning fork for testing vibration sensation (C_0 pitch).

Snellen chart 3m or 6m. Put this at a measured distance and make sure it is well-lit. Obtain a 'pin-hole on a stick' or make one.

Ophthalmoscope (If a team member has received appropriate training.) Working, with batteries, bulb, and a clean lens.

Tropicamide 0.5 or 1.0 per cent eye drops.

Urine testing kit Ketones; microalbumin and albumin.

Educational aids

- Essential leaflets from Diabetes UK: 'What is diabetes', 'What diabetes care to expect', and a diabetes diet leaflet
- A wide variety of other leaflets from Diabetes UK
- A finger-pricking device and lancets
- Blood glucose testing and urine testing strips
- An old insulin vial filled with water label 'demonstration only'
- Insulin syringes (0.5 ml and 1 ml) and needles
- A packet of tissues
- A sharps container
- A needle clipper
- Diabetes cards (Type 1 and Type 2)
- Medicalert and SOS literature
- A packet of Dextrosol or equivalent
- Larger diabetes clinics may stock demonstration insulin pens, cartridges filled with water, glucose meters, plastic foods, etc.

Hypoglycaemia kit

- Dextrose tablets and small bottles of Lucozade
- Hypostop gel
- Glucagon pack
- Tourniquet
- 2 intravenous cannulae
- Tape (e.g. micropore)
- 20 ml or 50 ml syringe
- 50 ml of 50 per cent dextrose × 2
- 2 × 10 ml ampoules 0.9 per cent saline (to flush dextrose through intravenous cannulae)
- Kettle, tea, milk, sugar, and a tin of biscuits (for both patients and staff)!

partner's patients. It is probably easier to set up a clinic but this takes protected time. A practice with 100 diabetic patients needs at least are full-session diabetic clinic a week.

As an approximate guide, and assuming that the patient spends half their time with the general practitioner and half their time with the practice nurse, a practice with 60 diabetic patients would need a session (i.e. a morning or an afternoon) a month to see each patient for about half an hour every six months. This does not include seeing new patients and does not provide adequate time for education for which an additional session a month (at least) should be set aside.

Organization

As patients need different things from different visits at different times, the patient and the staff need a record and reminder of what to do, when. A recall system retrieves patients for their annual review and identifies non-attenders. Patient-held records are useful only if the patient keeps them and brings them back each time, and the staff fill them in. There are several such records available. It is worth looking at what is available before going to the trouble and expense of designing your own. The person responsible for the diabetes register should also administer the clinic and organize appointment times etc. There are computer systems available but ensure that they are compatible with other surgery software and hardware and that they really do what you want. Unless you have a lot of people with diabetes it is not worth getting purpose-designed diabetes software.

Once the patients, the place, the staff, and the time have been organized, the process of care must be determined. Standards for the process and outcome of care should be determined and the method of audit should be considered. Audit should include identifying areas in which improvements are needed, feeding back the information, and making appropriate changes in care.

New patients

A practice with no previous experience of diabetes care should refer new patients to a diabetologist for initial assessment and management plan. Care thereafter can be agreed according to individual patient's needs.

Assessment

The details of areas to be covered on the first and subsequent examinations have been covered on the relevant chapters.

+ Confirm the diagnosis
+ Symptoms
+ Previous history (pancreatitis, autoimmune disease, cardiac disease, hypertension, surgery)
+ Obstetric history (gestational diabetes, big babies)
+ Family history (diabetes, autoimmune disease)
+ Smoking—STOP!
+ Alcohol (excess now or past?)
+ Drugs (thiazides, steroids)
+ Allergies (if allergic to sulphonamides do not give sulphonylureas)
+ Examination
+ Biochemistry (urea and electrolytes, creatinine, lipids)
+ Haematology (full blood count, HbA1$_c$).
+ Microbiology (pus or urine)
+ Consider ECG
+ Consider chest X-ray.

Education (see Chapter 4)

Survival
+ What diabetes is
+ What it means
+ Treatment—diet—reduce sugar
+ Treatment—hypoglycaemic therapy
+ How to monitor urine or blood glucose
+ Hypoglycaemia if relevant

Education (see Chapter 4) *(continued)*

- If driver, tell DVLA, motor insurance company
- Carry diabetes card
- Provide take-home literature
- Who to call for help
- Date and time of next appointment

Long term

- What diabetes is in detail
- What it means at home, work, and play
- What are the implications for the patient and his family, now and future?
- Diet in detail
- Exercise
- Blood glucose testing—treatment goals
- Details of oral hypoglycaemic treatment
- Details of insulin treatment and self-administration
- How to adjust treatment according to blood glucose
- Driving
- Body maintenance and preventive care
- Diabetes tissue damage
- Smoking
- Alcohol
- Travel
- Pregnancy and family planning

Examination

A full 'top-to-toe' clinical examination should be performed at diagnosis and at least every five years. Elderly patients and those with tissue damage may need more frequent examinations. The items below are especially relevant to diabetes and should form part of every initial and annual review. Those marked thus * should be checked on every attendance:

Physical

- Height (diagnosis only unless under 19 years old)
- Weight*
- Blood pressure* (lying and standing, annually)

- Feet—general appearance*
  —skin
  —evidence of infection
  —deformity
  —swelling
  —sensation (Monofilament)
  —pulses
- Legs—knee and ankle jerks
- Eyes—visual acuity
  —lens
  —retinae through dilated pupils if trained
  —or record results of formal diabetic eye check performed in accredited scheme
- Injection sites (insulin-treated patients)

Urine

- Albumin (microalbumin)
- Ketones

Blood

- Glucose*
- Glycosylated haemoglobin (* unless checked within 2 months)
- Creatinine
- Cholesterol and triglyceride (* if raised unless checked within 1 month)
- Thyroid function

Some authorities would check glycosylated haemoglobin and lipids more often if they are elevated.

Questions for every visit

- How are you? Home, work, play
- Any new concerns or problems?
- Glucose balance since last seen
- Evidence of hyperglycaemia

Questions for every visit (continued)

◆ Evidence of hypoglycaemia, warnings, help from others

◆ Diet

◆ Medication and any adverse effects

◆ Smoking if relevant

◆ Alcohol if relevant

◆ Family planning if relevant

◆ Diabetes educational needs

Who should be seen by whom?

Each patient should see their doctor, dietitian, chiropodist, and optometrist or ophthalmic optician annually.

General practitioners will have varying degrees of confidence in managing different patients and their problems. Ideally the patient should be able to move between specialist, general practitioner, and community services, gaining the best from each with the minimum of inconvenience, and perceiving no 'seams' between services.

Most general practitioners and diabetologists agree that children, teenagers, and pregnant women should be seen by diabetologists, as should patients with tissue damage and those with major instability of blood glucose balance. Agreements as to the arrangements for the shared care of such patients need to be made for each individual.

Many general practitioners wish to provide sole care for patients treated by diet alone and diet with tablets. Some are also happy to care for patients who have stable insulin-treated diabetes.

Audit

Several studies have audited diabetes care in general practice as compared with that of similar practices in the local hospital diabetes clinic. The Wolverhampton mini-clinic project was one of the earliest (Singh *et al.* 1984). Supported by an enthusiastic diabetologist, general practitioners managed patients with Type 1 and Type 2 diabetes. Patients were more likely to attend the mini-clinic (default rate 6 per cent), than the hospital (31 per cent), and their glycaemic balance was similar.

In Wales, Hayes and Harries (1984) also performed a randomized controlled trial of routine hospital clinic area versus routine general practice care for Type 2 diabetes. They included only those practices who wished to participate but did not provide any additional diabetes training for general practitioners. Patients under general practice care had higher glycosylated haemoglobin concentrations than those under hospital care. They were also more likely to die (GP care 18/103 died, hospital 6/97 died). The excess deaths appeared to be cardiovascular.

A review of the literature (Griffin and Kinmonth 2000) found five randomized trials in which patients were allocated to systematic diabetes review by primary care staff. Where specialist diabetes services provided intensive support and prompting for general practitioners and their patients, there was no difference in mortality between hospital and primary care, and HbA1 and default rates were lower in primary care. Where this support was not available mortality, follow-up, and HbA1 were worse in primary care. Diabetes education is essential for all staff caring for diabetic patients.

The Audit Commission (2000) in their report *Testing times* reviewed diabetes care nationally. In their audit they found that about 75 per cent of patients with diabetes were receiving routine care by primary care, but that a third of the clinics were run by practice nurses alone.

> A few years ago I had a telephone call from a practice nurse asking if she could see me urgently. When she arrived she was in a state of panic. 'My GP has asked me to run a diabetic clinic,' she said, nearly in tears, 'but I don't know anything about diabetes. He says I've got to do it. Please help me!' So we did.

Less than one third of practices had routine access to a dietitian or podiatrist. Over a third had no guidelines for referrals to specialists. One hospital diabetic foot clinic reported that half the patients had been referred late from the community.

Testing times highlighted the need for good communication across the primary/secondary care interface. They studied hospital notes and found that:

- ◆ one in five GP letters gave no clear indication of the problem that led to referral;
- ◆ one in four letters made no mention of current diabetes control;
- ◆ almost half of all letters failed to indicate what interim action had been taken by GPs;
- ◆ over two-thirds of records and letters from hospitals back to GPs failed to note what information had been given to the patient.

Patients were particularly concerned about waiting times in clinics and timing of appointments in hospitals, as compared with primary care clinics; although they had more concerns about written information and being able to get advice 'when I want it' in primary care.

The Audit Commission concluded that for diabetes care 'the solutions to coping with increased demands lie in primary care, supported by specialist diabetes teams'.

At the outset, establish a format for audit of the process and outcome of diabetes care (Table 21.1). Process measures include whether the items of clinical examination and urine/blood testing have been carried out, and whether the dietitian and chiropodist have been seen. Outcome measures include the findings on examination and urine/blood tests, as well as other measures of patient well-being and whether they are independent, for example. It should be noted that you can audit only what is recorded. Negative findings are valuable in diabetes care—it is good to know that there is no retinopathy or that the feet are normal. But if you do not write it down, no one will know that you checked it. Ideally, your diabetes record is also your audit form. It may be very difficult to extract the diabetes 'bits' from the rest of a bulky file and a separate record form is usually best.

Share the audit findings with the whole team and take steps to improve on less than perfect areas. Set realistic goals for next year. Share your experiences with other general practitioners and gain from theirs.

Table 21.1 Audit dataset* (Include all negative and normal data)

Patient identifier
Date of record
Date of birth, age
Sex
Year of diagnosis, duration of diabetes
Dead/alive
Pregnant
Treatment diet alone, tablets, insulin

Smoking
Alcohol

Appointments attended and missed

Weight, height, body mass index
Dietition seen, when
Glucose, HbA1$_c$/fructosamine
Injection sites
Hypoglycaemia requiring medical help/admission
Admissions for high glucose, ketoacidosis

Admissions, other e.g. heart
Admissions days
Sick days

Eyes—visual acuity, cataracts, retinopathy, eye treatment
Ophthalmologist seen, when

Feet—amputation, ulcer
Feet—monofilament
Symptomatic neuropathy (including non-foot)
Feet—pulses
Claudication, previous peripheral vascular disease
Chiropodist seen, when

BP systolic/diastolic
Creatinine, microalbumin, albumin
Renal dialysis/transplant

Cholesterol, triglycerides
Angina, myocardial infarct, previous ischaemic heart disease
Stroke, previous cerebrovascular disease

Impotence

Treatment—BP, angina, lipid, cardiac failuire

Education score
Well-being score
Satisfaction with service

* Wilson, A.E. and Home, P.D. (for the Diabetes Audit Working Group of the Research Unit of the Royal College of Physicians and the British Diabetic Association) (1993). A dataset to allow exchange of information for monitoring continuing diabetes care. *Diabetic Medicine*, 10, 378–90 (with modification).

Resources

Diabetes is a common, chronic, multisystem disease in which intensive preventive care and treatment have been shown to improve morbidity and mortality. The consequences of diabetes are costly.

The Cost of Diabetes in Europe—Type 2 (CODE-2) study (Williams *et al.* 2001) showed that in 749 patients in Bradford, Jersey, and Salford, during 1998, the management of each patient with Type 2 diabetes cost £1505 per annum. Thirty-six per cent of this cost was for hospital admissions, 38 per cent for ambulatory care, and 3 per cent for glucose-lowering drugs. Of those patients admitted to hospital, 82 per cent of the cost was related to diabetic complications. Assuming a prevalence of diabetes of 2 per cent (an underestimation nowadays), the authors estimated that the total NHS cost of Type 2 diabetes is £1.8 billion—4.1 per cent of the total expenditure on the NHS. Figures like this were found in other European countries. The main costs of diabetes complications relate to secondary care. In one district general hospital on one day in 2000, nearly 10 per cent of all in-patients had diabetes. With good preventive care the numbers and length of such admissions could be reduced over time. For Type 2 diabetes, the authors of UKPDS calculated in 1998 (UKPDS 40) that the additional resources required to achieve tight blood pressure control were £261 to £720 per year of life gained. This compares very favourably with costs for preventive care in other conditions.

Summary

- When establishing a diabetes service in primary care find out how many patients to expect, how many you actually have, and what resources are required.

- Resources include accommodation, staff, training, experience, time, and equipment.

- Plan the clinic organization, records, and audit.

- Follow the management protocols and modify them to suit your patients.*

- Audit what you are doing and the outcomes.

- Feed back audit findings to improve your service.

References and further reading

Audit Commission (2000). *Testing times: a review of diabetes services in England and Wales.* (Obtainable via telephone 0800 502030) (See also *www.diabetes.audit-commission.gov.uk*)

Greenhalgh, T. (ed) (1998). Diabetes care: a primary care perspective. *Diabetic Medicine*, 15, Suppl. 3.

Griffin, S., and Kinmonth, A.L. (2000). Diabetes care: the effectiveness of systems for routine surveillance for people with diabetes. *Cochrane Database of Systemic Review* (2): CD 000541.

Hayes, T.M., and Harries, J. (1984). Randomised controlled trial of routine hospital clinic care versus routine general practice care for Type II diabetics. *British Medical Journal*, 289, 728.

Porter, A.M.D. (1982). Organisation of diabetic care. *British Medical Journal*, 285, 1121.

Singh, B.M., Holland, M.R., Thorn, P.A., *et al.* (1984). Metabolic control of diabetes in general practice clinics—comparison with a hospital clinic. *British Medical Journal*, 289, 726–8.

UK Prospective Diabetes Study Group (1998). Cost effectiveness analysis of improved blood pressure control in hypertensive patients with type 2 diabetes: UKPDS 40. *British Medical Journal*, 317, 720–6.

Williams, R., *et al.* (2001). CODE-2 UK: our contribution to a European study of the costs of type 2 diabetes. *Practical Diabetes International*, 18, 235–8.

* An example of one district's guidelines for aspects of diabetes management in primary care—'The Hillingdon Consensus Care Diabetes Project' is shown in Appendix A (p. 211).

Chapter 22

Diabetes charters

St Vincent Declaration

Representatives of Government Health Departments and patients' organizations from all European countries met with diabetes experts under the aegis of the Regional Offices of the World Health Organisation (WHO) and the International Diabetes Federation (IDF) in St Vincent, Italy on October 10–12, 1989. They unanimously agreed upon the following recommendations and urged that they should be presented in all countries throughout Europe for implementation.

Diabetes mellitus is a major and growing European health problem, a problem at all ages and in all countries. It causes prolonged ill-health and early death. It threatens at least ten million European citizens.

It is within the power of national Governments and Health Departments to create conditions in which a major reduction in this heavy burden of disease and death can be achieved. Countries should give formal recognition to the diabetes problem and deploy resources for its solution. Plans for the prevention, identification and treatment of diabetes and particularly its complications—blindness, renal failure, gangrene and amputation, aggravated coronary heart disease and stroke—should be formulated at local, national and European regional levels. Investment now will earn great dividends in reduction of human misery and in massive savings of human and material resources.

General goals and five-year targets listed below can be achieved by the organized activities of the medical services in active partnership with diabetic citizens, their families, friends, and workmates and their organizations; in the management of their own diabetes and the education for it; in the planning, provision, and quality audit of health care; in national, regional, and international organizations for disseminating information about health maintenance; in promoting and applying research.

General goals for people—children and adults—with diabetes

- Sustained improvement in health experience and a life approaching normal in expectation in quality and quantity.

- Prevention and cure of diabetes and of its complications by intensifying research effort.

Five-year targets

Elaborate, initiate, and evaluate comprehensive programmes for detection and control of diabetes and of its complications with self-care and community support as major components.

Raise awareness in the population and among health care professionals of the present opportunities and the future needs for prevention of the complications of diabetes and of diabetes itself.

Organize training and teaching in diabetes management and care for people of all ages with diabetes, for their families, friends, and working associates and for the health care team.

Ensure that care for children with diabetes is provided by individuals and teams specialized both in the management of diabetes and of children, and that families with a diabetic child get the necessary social, economic, and emotional support.

Reinforce existing centres of excellence in diabetes care, education and research. Create new centres where the need and potential exist.

Promote independence, equity, and self-sufficiency for all people with diabetes—children, adolescents, those in the working years of life and the elderly.

Remove hindrances to the fullest possible integration of the diabetic citizen into society.

Implement effective measures for the prevention of costly complications:

◆ Reduce new blindness due to diabetes by one-third or more.

◆ Reduce numbers of people entering end-stage diabetic renal failure by at least one-third.

◆ Cut morbidity and mortality from coronary heart disease in the diabetic by vigorous programmes of risk factor reduction.

◆ Achieve pregnancy outcome in the diabetic woman that approximates to that of the non-diabetic woman.

Establish monitoring and control systems using state-of-the-art information technology for quality assurance of diabetes health care provision and for laboratory and technical procedures in diabetes diagnosis, treatment, and self-management.

Promote European and international collaboration in programmes of diabetes research and development through national, regional, and WHO agencies and in active partnership with diabetes patient organizations.

Take urgent action in the spirit of the WHO programme 'Health for all' to establish joint machinery between WHO and International Diabetes Federation, European Region, to initiate, accelerate, and facilitate the implementation of the recommendations.

The European Patients' Charter

In 1991 the European Region of the International Diabetes Federation and the St Vincent Steering Committee at the WHO Europe produced the first charter for people with diabetes in Europe.

Your guide to better diabetes care: rights and roles

A person with diabetes can, in general, lead a normal, healthy and long life. Looking after yourself (self-care) by learning about your diabetes provides the best chance to do this. Your doctor and the other members of the health care team (made up of doctor(s), nurses, dietitian(s), chiropodist(s)) are there to advise you and to provide the information, support, and technology so that you can look after yourself, and live your life in the way you choose.

It is important that you should know:

1 what should be available from your health providers to help you reach these goals;

2 what *you* should do.

Your rights

The health care team (providers) should provide:

- a treatment plan and self-care targets;
- regular checks of blood sugar (glucose) levels and of your physical condition;
- treatment of special problems and emergencies;
- continuing education for you and your family;
- information on available social and economic support.

Your role is:

- to build this advice into your daily life; and
- to be in control of your diabetes on a day-to-day basis.

Continuing education

The following are important items you should learn about:

1 Why it is necessary to control blood glucose levels.
2 How to control your blood glucose levels through proper eating, physical activity, tablets, and/or insulin.
3 How to monitor your control with blood or urine tests (self-monitoring) and how to act on the results.
4 The signs of low and high blood glucose levels and ketosis, how to prevent them, and how to treat them.
5 What to do when you are ill.
6 The possible long-term complications—including possible damage to eyes, nerves, kidneys, and feet, and hardening of the arteries; their prevention and their treatment.
7 How to deal with lifestyle variations such as exercise, travelling, and social activities including drinking alcohol.
8 How to handle possible problems with employment, insurance, driving licences, etc.

Treatment plan and self-care targets

The following should be given to you:

1 Personalized advice on proper eating—types of food, amount and timing.
2 Advice on physical activity.
3 Your dose and timing of tablets or insulin—and how to take them; advice on how to change doses based on your self-monitoring.
4 Your target values for blood glucose, blood fats, blood pressure, and weight.

Regular checks

The following should be done **at each visit** to your health care professionals: (NB these may vary according to your particular needs)

1 Review of your self-monitoring results and current treatment.

2 Talk about your targets and change where necessary.

3 Talk about any problems and questions you may have.

4 Continued education.

The **health care team** should check:

1 Your blood glucose control by taking special blood tests, such as HbA1 or fructosamine (fasting blood glucose in non-insulin-treated people); this can be done two to four times per year if your diabetes is well controlled.

2 Your weight.

3 Your blood pressure and blood fats, if necessary.

The following should be checked at least **once per year:**

1 Your eyes and vision.

2 Your kidney function (blood and urine tests).

3 Your feet.

4 Your risk factors for heart disease, such as blood pressure, blood fats, and smoking habits.

5 Your self-monitoring and injection techniques.

6 Your eating habits.

Special situations

1 Advice and care should be available if you are planning to become or are pregnant.

2 The needs of children and adolescents should be cared for.

3 If you have problems with eyes, kidneys, feet, blood vessels or heart, then you should be able to see specialists quickly.

4 In the elderly, strict treatment is often unnecessary. You may want to discuss this with your health care team.

5 The first months after your diabetes has been discovered are often difficult. Remember you cannot learn everything during this period—learning will continue for the rest of your life.

6 You should receive clear information on what to do in emergencies.

Your role

◆ To take control of your diabetes on a day-to-day basis. This will be easier the more you know about your diabetes.

◆ Learn about and practise self-care. This includes monitoring glucose levels and how to change your treatment according to the results.

◆ To examine your feet regularly.

- Follow good lifestyle practices: these include choosing the right food, weight control, regular physical activity, and not smoking.
- Know when to contact your health care team urgently, including for emergencies.
- Regularly talk with your health care team about questions and concerns you may have.
- Ask questions—and repeat them if you are still unclear. Prepare your questions beforehand.
- Speak to your health care team, other people with diabetes, and your local or national Diabetes Association and read the pamphlets and books about diabetes provided by your health care team or diabetes association. Make sure your family and friends know about the needs of your diabetes.

If you feel that adequate facilities and care are not available to help you look after your diabetes then contact your local or national Diabetes Association.

National Service Framework (NSF)

The Diabetes NSF is still awaited although standards have been published and can be viewed on *www.doh.gov.uk/nsf/diabetes.*

Appendix A: Hillingdon Consensus Care Diabetes Project Guidelines

Reproduced from the Hillingdon Consensus Care Diabetes Project 2001 (Chair Dr Rowan Hillson) with permission. No part of these Hillingdon Consensus Care Diabetes Guidelines may be reproduced without permission.

Reducing Risk Factors
Summary Sheet

Risk Factor	Action	Aim
Smoking	STOP	No Smoking
Hypertension	*Treat with:* ACE Inhibitor Bendrofluazide Beta Blocker Calcium Channel Blocker	BP below 130/80 (<125/75 if proteinuria) Beware postural drop
High Glucose	*Treat with:* Diabetic Diet Sulphonylurea Metformin Insulin	4–6 mmol/l fasting 4–8 mmol/l rest of time HbA1$_c$ 4.5–6.4% Avoid hypoglycaemia
High Cholesterol	*Treat with:* Low fat diet Statin Fibrate	Below 5mmol/l
Myocardial infarct	*Treat with:* Aspirin Statin Beta Blocker ACE Inhibitor Insulin	No further events

Reducing Hypertension
Important : Refer to Cardiology Care Guidelines

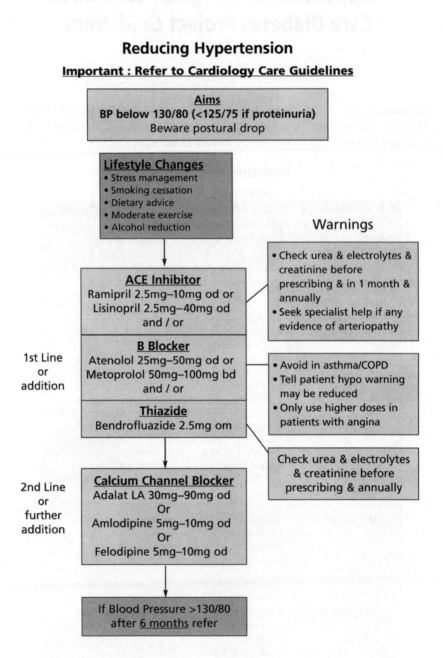

Aims
BP below 130/80 (<125/75 if proteinuria)
Beware postural drop

Lifestyle Changes
• Stress management
• Smoking cessation
• Dietary advice
• Moderate exercise
• Alcohol reduction

Warnings

1st Line or addition

ACE Inhibitor
Ramipril 2.5mg–10mg od or
Lisinopril 2.5mg–40mg od
and / or

• Check urea & electrolytes & creatinine before prescribing & in 1 month & annually
• Seek specialist help if any evidence of arteriopathy

B Blocker
Atenolol 25mg–50mg od or
Metoprolol 50mg–100mg bd
and / or

Thiazide
Bendrofluazide 2.5mg om

• Avoid in asthma/COPD
• Tell patient hypo warning may be reduced
• Only use higher doses in patients with angina

2nd Line or further addition

Calcium Channel Blocker
Adalat LA 30mg–90mg od
Or
Amlodipine 5mg–10mg od
Or
Felodipine 5mg–10mg od

Check urea & electrolytes & creatinine before prescribing & annually

If Blood Pressure >130/80
after 6 months refer

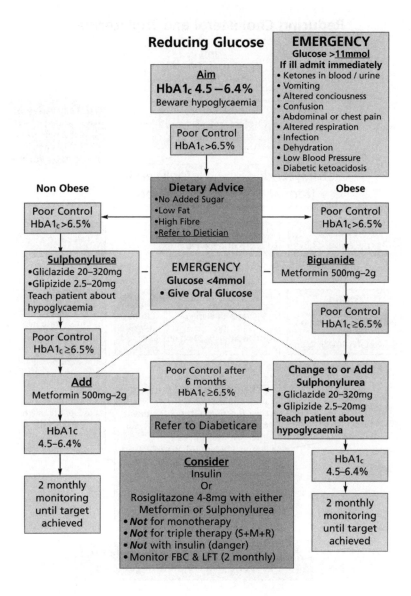

Reducing Glucose

EMERGENCY
Glucose >11mmol
If ill admit immediately
• Ketones in blood / urine
• Vomiting
• Altered conciousness
• Confusion
• Abdominal or chest pain
• Altered respiration
• Infection
• Dehydration
• Low Blood Pressure
• Diabetic ketoacidosis

Aim
HbA1c 4.5 – 6.4%
Beware hypoglycaemia

Poor Control
HbA1c >6.5%

Non Obese

Obese

Poor Control
HbA1c >6.5%

Dietary Advice
•No Added Sugar
•Low Fat
•High Fibre
•Refer to Dietician

Poor Control
HbA1c >6.5%

Sulphonylurea
•Gliclazide 20–320mg
•Glipizide 2.5–20mg
Teach patient about
hypoglycaemia

EMERGENCY
Glucose <4mmol
• Give Oral Glucose

Biguanide
Metformin 500mg–2g

Poor Control
HbA1c ≥6.5%

Poor Control
HbA1c ≥6.5%

Add
Metformin 500mg–2g

Poor Control after
6 months
HbA1c ≥6.5%

**Change to or Add
Sulphonylurea**
• Gliclazide 20–320mg
• Glipizide 2.5–20mg
Teach patient about
hypoglycaemia

HbA1c
4.5–6.4%

Refer to Diabeticare

2 monthly
monitoring
until target
achieved

Consider
Insulin
Or
Rosiglitazone 4-8mg with either
Metformin or Sulphonylurea
• *Not* for monotherapy
• *Not* for triple therapy (S+M+R)
• *Not* with insulin (danger)
• Monitor FBC & LFT (2 monthly)

HbA1c
4.5–6.4%

2 monthly
monitoring
until target
achieved

Reducing Cholesterol and Triglyceride

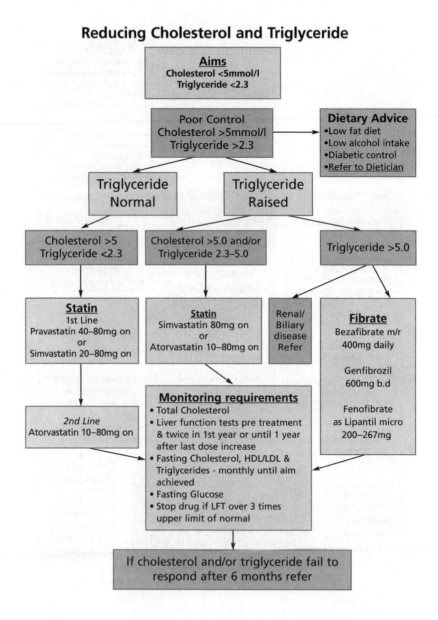

Primary Care Annual Review

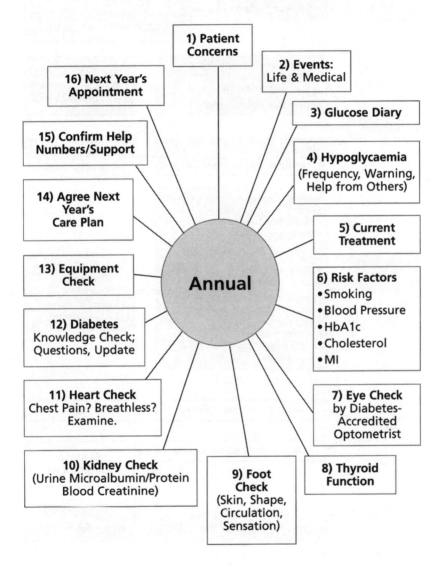

Complication Check

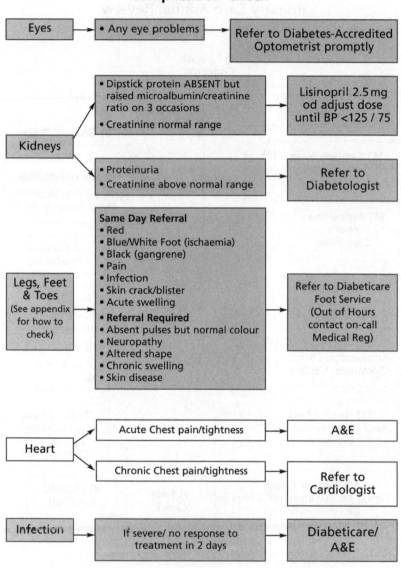

Diabetes in Hillingdon
Referral letter

Date of appointment   Date of referral

To: Diabeticare   From:
The Hillingdon Hospital
Uxbridge
Middlesex UB8 3NN
(T) 01895 279265 (F) 01895 279521   (T)   (F)

Name	Date of birth	Age
Address	NHS number	
	Hospital number	
Telephone (day)	(night)	Mobile
Occupation		

Date of diagnosis of diabetes		**Family history** yes / no	
Symptoms thirst/polyuria/weight loss		**Other**	
Complications			
Coronary dis.	Periph. vasc. dis.	Stroke/TIA	Hypertension
Retinopathy	Cataract	Neuropathy	Nephropathy
Skin problem/ulcer	Foot problem	Infection	Ketoacidosis Hypo

Other medical history

Smoker	yes/no	Alcohol	units/week		Driver? yes / no	
Weight		Height	BP		Urine dip	
Diagnostic glucose		Fasting	Random/2hr		HbA1c	
Chol.	Trig.	FT4	TSH	Hb	WBC	Plts
Na K U	Creatinine	Bilirubin	ALT	AlkPhos	Albumin	

Treatment	**Allergies**
Signed	

Diabetes in Hillingdon **Your name**

Consensus Care **Date**

Questions for people with diabetes
Please fill in this form before you see your doctor or nurse. It is to help check how you and your diabetes are getting on.

Changes? New surname / address / phone number? Please note it here:

Do you drive? Yes / no

Have you been to hospital in the past year?
(as an in-patient or out-patient) With what?

How is your blood glucose? Don't forget to bring your record.
(OK, too high, too low?)

Have you had low sugar reactions (hypoglycaemic episode)?
Yes / no
Did you know it was happening?
Did you need help?

Have you had any of the following:

Problems with your vision	Yes / no	Soreness of vagina / penis	Yes / no
Chest pain or discomfort	Yes / no	Breathlessness	Yes / no
Problems with your feet	Yes / no	Foot rubs / blisters / cracks	Yes / no
Change in foot / toe colour	Yes / no	Foot pain	Yes / no
Tingling in hands or feet	Yes / no	Numbness in hands or feet	Yes / no
Thirst	Yes / no	Passing urine more often	Yes / no

Have you any questions you want to ask?

SCREENING FOR THE AT RISK DIABETIC FOOT IN GENERAL PRACTICE

Guide to the use of Monofilaments for sensory testing on the foot

1 Use the 10g monofilament to test sensation.

2 The sites to be tested are indicated on the foot diagram below.

3 Apply the filament perpendicular to the skin's surface (see Diagram A).

4 The approach, skin contact and departure of the monofilament should be approximately 1.5 seconds duration.

5 Apply sufficient force to allow the filament to bend (see Diagram B).

6 Do not allow the filament to slide across the skin or make repetitive contact at the test site.

7 Randomise the order and timing of successive tests (to reduce potential for patient guessing).

8 Ask the patient to respond 'yes' when the filament is felt.

9 Do not apply to an ulcer site, callous, scar or necrotic tissue.

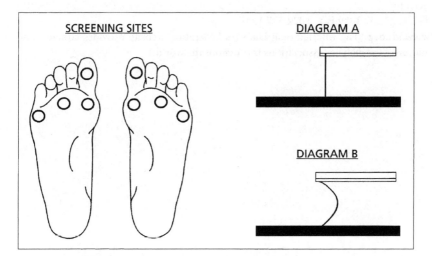

Consider the patient's feet to be 'at risk' if the patient cannot feel the 10gm monofilament at any of the sites marked.

Appendix B: Diabetes associations

Diabetes UK,
10, Parkway,
London, NW1 7AA
Tel. 020 7424 1000 Fax. 020 7424 1001
www.diabetes.org.uk

European Association for the Study of Diabetes,
Rheindorfer Weg 3,
D-40591,
Dusseldorf,
Germany
Tel. +49 211 75 84 69 0 Fax. +49 211 75 84 69 29
www.easd.org

International Diabetes Federation
1 rue Defacqz
B-1000 Brussels
Belgium
Tel. +322 537 1889 Fax. +322 537 1981
www.idf.org (The International Diabetes Federation website provides contacts and addresses for diabetes associations throughout the world.)

Appendix C: Useful contacts

- Audit Commission
  www.diabetes.audit-commission.gov.uk

- British Hypertension Society
  www.hyp.ac.uk/bhs

- Children with diabetes
  www.childrenwithdiabetes.com/index_cwd.htm

- Diabetes Discrimination in Employment
  www.users.globalnet.co.uk/%7Eifduk

- Diabetes Insight
  www.diabetic.org.uk

- Diabetes Monitor
  www.diabetesmonitor.com

- Diabetes Network International
  www.dni.org.uk

- Diabetic Medicine On-line
  www.blackwell-science.com/dme

- European Association for the Study of Diabetic Eye Complications
  www.diabeticretinopathy.org.uk

- Insulin Pumpers UK
  www.insulin-pumpers.org.uk

- National Institute for Clinical Excellence (NICE)
  www.nice.org.uk

- National Service Framework for Diabetes
  www.doh.gov.uk/nsf/diabetes

These websites contain information about diabetes and related issues. The accuracy of this information has not been checked and Dr Hillson does not endorse or accept responsibility for websites shown in this book.

Appendix D: Books

For people with diabetes

Diabetes UK publish leaflets on most diabetes topics. Some can be downloaded from their website. They also provide lists of books written for people with diabetes. One such book, consistent with *Practical Diabetes Care* is: Rowan Hillson (2002). *Diabetes: the complete guide* (3rd edn). Vermilion, Ebury Press, London.

Reference books

Alberti, K.G.M.M. (1997). *International textbook of diabetes mellitus*. John Wiley, Chichester.
Pickup, J. and Williams, G. (1996). *Textbook of diabetes*. Blackwell Science, Oxford.

Index